The Complete

Fasting Guide

To Miraculous Health

And Well-Being

How to Be Thinner, Happier And
More Energetic Through Healthy
Fasting

By

Jillian Bradley

☒

ISBN-13: 978-1475155044

Table of Contents

Introduction

Fad diets don't work. Do you want
to *play* at weight loss, or take
control and lose weight?

I'm not going to kid you. Weight loss for most people is hard.
Duh! Take a look around at our obese society. They're
everywhere. At every economic and social level. In every ethnic
group and color. In every religion and at every age. We are one,
big nation of fat-bodies.

And *lay-zee...* Why are we so fat? Because it's too hard to push
ourselves away from that fast-food table and too hard to get up
and do something physical. So we go on that fad diet we heard
about on TV. You know, the one that's got *all* of Hollywood
talking. And guess what. It doesn't work either. Why?

Because no one wants to put forth the effort it takes to actually
lose weight. Read that again - *because no one wants to put forth
the effort it takes to actually lose weight.* Did you get that? And
it's really ironic, as well, because there are only two rules to
weight loss: (1) eat less and (2) exercise more. Why do we have
to make it so hard? *Eat less and exercise more!*

How many of these 'fad' diets have you tried?

> Low-carb diet
> Acai berry diet
> Negative calorie diet
> Apple cider vinegar diet

Low-fat diet
Grapefruit diet
Macrobiotic diet
All meat diet
Cabbage soup diet

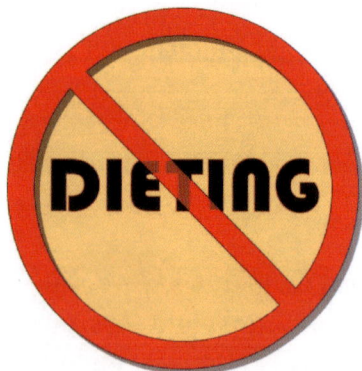

How many have worked? The truth about virtually *all* of the fad diets is they don't help to lose weight and keep the weight off. I mean think about it: if a fad diet really worked, everyone would be on it and stay on it.

The *only* way to effectively lose weight is to take in fewer calories then you are expending during the day. But no one wants to hear that. Why? Because (1) we love to eat (2) we hate to exercise and (3) we lack the self-discipline *to change* to a healthier life *style.*

If you're not serious about weight-loss and a lifetime of self-control over your health and well being, then this book will not benefit you one bit. But if you do want to lose weight, change your eating and exercise habits in a way that has been proven by millions of people the world over and for over 7,000 years, then *The Complete Fasting Guide To Miraculous Health And Well-Being* will start you on a journey that will change you forever.

Are you tired of looking into the mirror and seeing a fat-person staring back? Do you want to look good in that summer bikini? Would you like to turn heads again? Do you want to fit that into dress or tuxedo for your wedding? Do you want to quit breathing so hard just moving around? Then *The Complete Fasting Guide To Miraculous Health And Well-Being will* help you.

I have taught and practiced Guerrilla Weight Loss for over 32 years. Whenever I am participating, I lose a pound of fat a day.

For as long as I stay with it – *one pound every of fat and toxic body poisons every day. The Complete Fasting Guide To Miraculous Health And Well-Being* is not a diet or program. It is a lifestyle change. A radical one. And it has afforded me – and others - a wholesome, healthy lifestyle, physically, mentally and spiritually. You will lose weight and you will keep it off.

Recent studies since 2009 have shown that it takes most people 66 days to form a new habit. By habit, I mean that the behavior becomes 'as automatic as it is going to ever be' in 66 days. And *fasting* is no different. By learning the why's, how's, when's and how often and then putting them consciously in to practice, after about 66 days your life will have changed dramatically for the better and it will become a habit.

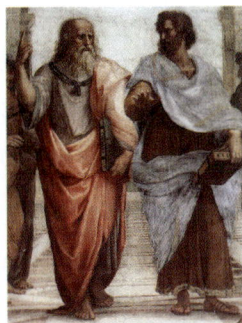

Fasting is simple: Eat less and exercise more. Fasting is an institution as old as Adam. Plato, the Greek philosopher of the 5th century B.C. said, "I fast for greater physical and mental efficiency."

Are you overweight, in need of dramatically losing a few (or several) pounds of unwanted fat *without* all the hype of fad dieting? Are your thoughts clouded and dull? Is your memory slow and fading? Is your spirit tired, emotionally drained and stressed? Has the skip gone out of your step? Are you plagued by numbing, poor health that you just can't put your finger on? Or have you simply lost your overall sense of well being?

Then fast and exercise.

I imagine at this point you must be thinking, 'But how do I fast?' 'Is fasting safe?' 'What are the benefits of fasting, and what are the concerns?' If you answered, "yes" to any one of the issues above, and have these same questions or more about fasting, then *The Complete Fasting Guide to Miraculous Health and Well-Being* is the book that will answer all of your questions.

Inside this book you will find information on:

1) What exactly *is* fasting?
2) Fasting for weight loss
3) Benefits of fasting
4) Fasting tips
5) Fasting with *only* water
6) Juice fasting and detoxification
7) Various fasting durations
8) Fasting safely
9) Fasting and detoxification recipes
10) How to safely *stop* fasting
11) Who can fast and who shouldn't
12) Fasting for your physical, mental, spiritual and emotional health

13) *And more*!

Whether you are an experienced faster or are completely new and seriously committed to the dramatic benefits you will experience by fasting, *The Complete Fasting Guide To Miraculous Health And Well-Being* will enlighten, entertain and educate you throughout your entire adventure.

There's an old adage, 'food is life.' Well, if food is life, then fasting is 'life on steroids!'

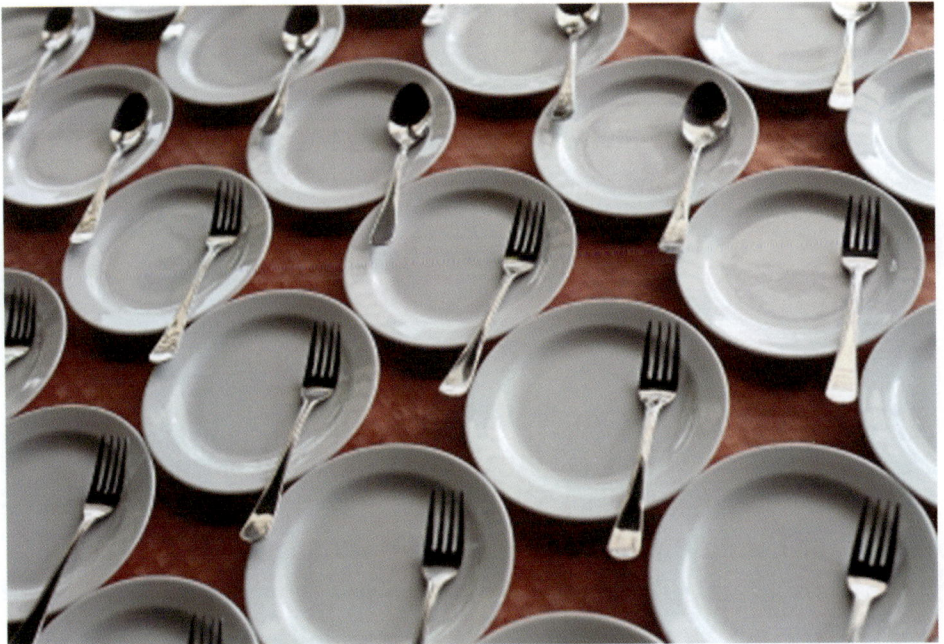

The Miracles of Fasting Proven Throughout History

What exactly is fasting?

Fasting is not a fad. Fasting in its simplest form is the cleansing abstinence from food. It is either fully avoiding eating anything or, in some cases, giving up *certain* foods, such as meat. Juice fasting allows for liquid teas, fruit and vegetable diets but no chewable food. A more aggressive fast may involve renouncing anything except water, as well. Juices, teas and other non-water drinks are avoided entirely, as well as food. Extreme *dry* fasting eliminates everything – food and water.

Fasting should not be confused with a vegan or vegetarian lifestyle, however. The effects and benefits of each may be similar, but the motivations and goals are completely different.

Of course, there are several variations in between, from extreme 'dry' and 'water-only fasting' to more liberal juice fasts and even abstinence from only certain – but not all - foods. The kind of fast you undertake will depend on your overall health, needs and goals as well as your physician's guidance for more depriving fasts.

Where did fasting originate?

Fasting, in various forms, is an old practice. People in virtually every culture, religion and ethnic class fasted. Men, women and even children historically participated in fasts. Christian, Buddhist, Hindu, Muslim, Judaism and virtually all major religions practiced fasting as a way to purify their carnal natures, gain self-discipline and regain closeness to their God. Throughout history and even in modern times, men and women were slaves to their bodies, needs and desires. So fasting also served as a way to discipline, or gain control, over their individual will power, habits and bodies.

Many of society's educated men and women considered the healing benefits of fasting as essential and regular activities in their own lives. In Chinese history, fasts were an important part of preventive medicine. Historically, doctors regularly required patients to fast in order to cleanse their bodies of impurities and toxins, restoring them to stasis. These same physicians practiced what they preached. They participated in their own therapeutic fasts for exactly the same healing benefits they proposed that their patients undergo. Philosophers experienced clearer thinking, deeper concentration and heightened awareness of life and the environment around them. Scientists in almost every discipline fasted to improve their memories, their abilities to reason and concentrate and to just plain 'think.'

These elite, as well as the myriad of lay-folks all knew and understood that one of the most powerfully designed tools for a healthy existence was *fasting.* And it was therefore, a significant part of their lives and living experiences.

But as time and the centuries pass, fasting – for whatever reason – has gone out of vogue and has become lost in modern circles and practices.

What happened to good, old-fashioned fasting?

We live in a fast paced, hurry up, '*go, go, go,*' stressed-out, consequents-be-damned world. We don't eat right yet we live to eat. So we gain weight and have become an obese society. Then we crash on another fad-diet and we don't eat right yet again – a vicious and dangerous circle. We pop pills to lose weight. Pills to stay awake and pills to go to sleep. We're undernourished *and* over-nourished. Our bodies bulge with fat so we go to a cosmetic surgeon to have the stuff sucked out or stapled shut or knots tied in our stomachs. After which, the cycle of eat, gain and *radically* reduce usually goes around and repeats itself again and again and again. We hate looking into a mirror, because there's a fat person staring back. We're stressed and on edge, and angry; we can't think straight, can't remember anything, have no energy and waning motivation. Something's always wrong with us, but we just can't quite put our finger on what's the problem. We can't exercise, we can't think and our romance and sex lives suffer. But hey! Another pill's *gotta help*!

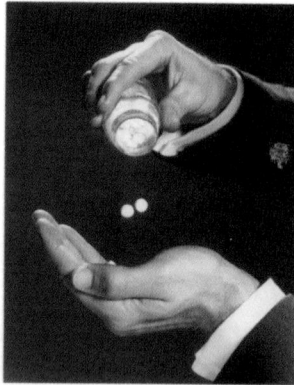

Along the way, we forgot the valuable 'whole-health' benefits that fasting provides. Something as simple as saying, 'no' to food; that which not only sustains us, but enslaves us, as well.

The ancients *knew* the value of fasting. They *knew* the healing benefits. They *knew* that saying, 'no' to one, three or seven days' of meals was *so much easier* and healthier than trying to lose weight (they actually had no concept of 'dieting.') Feeling better in every way in the long run was worth the short-term sacrifice. So they fasted.

The origins of diets and dieting

The earliest forms of a 'diet' or 'dieting' were found in B.C. Greek culture and the earliest Christian times. The language used from the Greek word 'diaita' meaning *prescribed way of living* (and therefor the practice) was related to *fasting.* It wasn't in any way like our fad diets of modern times.

In the 18th Century, the term 'diet' came to mean 'food' or 'rations' that were served in penal institutions, prisons and jailhouses. 'Bread and water' was a diet. A ration of cheese and

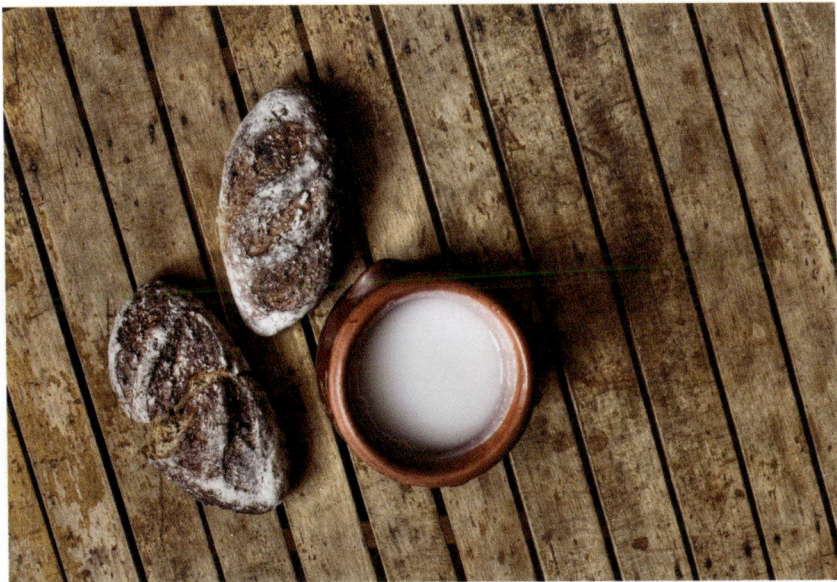

crackers was a 'diet.' Maybe that's why today, dieting is such an awful, painful regimen. It was meant for prisoners and inmates!

In all actuality, dieting as we have come to know the process didn't even come in to vogue until late in the 19th Century.

Historians generally agree that in 1863, a London undertaker, William Banting (1797 – 1878) decided he needed to lose his *fat-body*. He composed a pamphlet called *Letter on Corpulence, Addressed to the Public.* A doctor had offered him the following advice, and Mr. Banting created the first, 'fad diet':

1) Eat up to four meals everyday and each should include protein, some greens, fruits and 'a dry wine.'
2) Try to avoid starches and sugars
3) It's ok to have milk, butter and meat

William Banting lost 46 pounds in 12 months and we've been dieting ever since.

Prior to this event, people *fasted.* The masses didn't have the luxury of gorging themselves on food and drink, thereby gaining unnecessary weight. Being obese was limited to royalty and aristocrats.

Fasting is still valid in the 21st Century

There is virtually no other healing process that has been around for over 7,000 years, yet is still valid and proven to be just as successful as a modern-day practice as it was eons ago. The institution of fasting isn't dead; it's very much alive. It is often, however, simply misunderstood.

Today, probably more than at any other time in history, fasting is extremely relevant for our lives. The overall benefits of a fast actually fit very well with the stressful, unhappy, disillusioned and fast-paced lives we live today. Fasting fills the bill where time is at a premium and results need to be realized quickly. In almost every way, fasting will move us from obese to thin and from thin to healthy. From stressed to peaceful and from worry and anger to calm and peace. It will cleanse us of the toxins slowly poisoning our beings. And it can refresh our mental alertness, restore our waning energies and fuel our spiritual well being.

Lose Weight, Gain More Energy and Be Happier - The Health Benefits of Fasting

"Fasting cleanses the soul, raises the mind, subjects one's flesh to the spirit, renders the heart contrite and humble, scatters the clouds of concupiscence, quenches the fire of lust, and kindles the true light of chastity. Enter again into yourself." – Saint Augustine (3354-430 A.D.); *On Prayer and Fasting*, Sermon lxxii

Fasting advantages at a glance

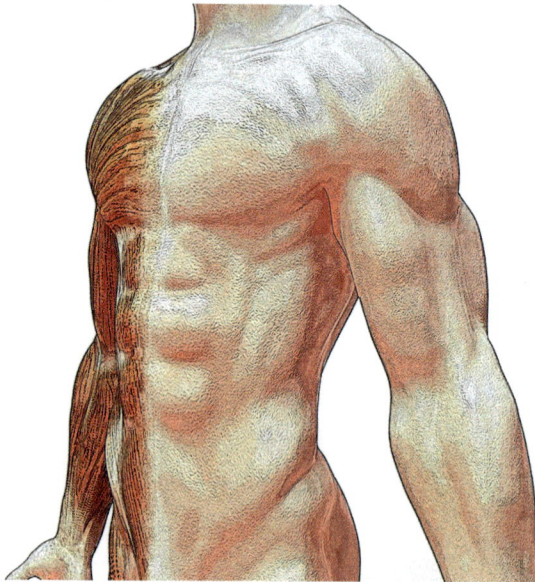

When participating in a fast, virtually every part of your being profits: your spirit, your body and your mental and emotional states. Almost universally, and with every individual, these benefits are, to some degree, the same. Let's take a more in-depth look at specific, positive health contributions realized from fasting. Right off the top of my head, some benefits include:

Loss of weight
Lower blood pressure
Delays the onset of age-related diseases such as
Alzheimer's and diabetes
Has been linked to the prevention of heart disease
Cleanses the poisonous toxins from your body
Physically repairs your body
Eliminates or reduces allergies
Gives you mental clarity
Facilitates restful sleep
Actually contributes to a longer life

What happens to you physiologically when you fast?

As soon as a fast begins, there is no longer any outside nourishment being introduced into the body to be processed in to energy or fuel. A process called *autolysis* begins which simply means that the body recognizes there is no fuel coming in so it begins to turn to its own internal resources to compensate the body's energy needs. The fat stores are converted by the liver and kidneys in to energy (fuel) and distributed throughout the body via the circulatory system. Ketone bodies, the water-soluble compounds produced as a by-product of this fatty acid-to-energy conversion are produced; a process called *ketosis*. The less fuel coming in means the more ketone bodies are created and used to keep up with the body's energy needs. Ketones are made up of three dissolved substances, two of which fuel the brain and heart. The third is simply a waste product that eventually gets excreted from the body.

When in a fasting state, a portion of the brain's energy comes from the water-soluble ketone bodies, as less glucose is available. The brain does not have any energy sources besides the body's glucose stores, unbound medium-chain fatty acids, which are soluble in the blood and these ketones. Within three days, the brain gets 25% of its energy from ketones. After roughly 40 days, ketone bodies fuel 70% of the brain's requirements. By now, the body's glucose stores are nearly completely exhausted.

Your body ingests toxins all the time in every meal you eat, every drink and every breath you take. And just as your heart beats and your lungs breathe, your body detoxifies. Additionally, in our modern society you are *inundated* with environmental poisons and toxins that your body doesn't know *how* to eliminate. So it stores them in your body's fatty deposits so you aren't poisoned.

Although your body detoxifies every single day, *serious* detoxification is initiated within the first 24-hours of beginning to fast. When your body realizes it needs energy but isn't being fed its normal, external fuel, your skin, lymph glands, colon, lungs, liver, kidneys and other organs all begin eliminating the toxins your body has gathered and stored over time. As your body fat now becomes the energy source, the toxins begin to radically burn away and are eliminated.

While your body is in a fasting state and no longer receiving external sources of fuel, it turns inward and looks at its own resources for energy. But everything your body creates or stores is not a *valuable* source of fuel. Your body, for example, does not properly nor adequately sustain benign tumors or abnormal growths. So, these become some of the first internal abnormalities susceptible to autolysis – and the first to become waste products and dissipate.

Of course, there are many other physiological changes that occur during fasting. Your body's core temperature drops, because metabolism and general overall bodily functions slows. Your body goes into this sort of 'hibernation state' to conserve as much of the internal energy sources as possible.

Growth and anti-aging hormones are released into your system. Energy during fasting is diverted away from your digestive system to the immune system, where healing begins to occur. It has been well studied and documented that under-nourishment – without malnourishment – actually extends life. Experiments on earthworms have been performed that, if translated to humans longevity, could extend the life of a man for 600-700 years. Fasting has been associated with the delay of age-related problems such as heart disease, Alzheimer's and diabetes.

Whew! That was a mouthful (ha-ha, so to speak...) but what does all this mean to you?

In short, fasting has been proven to heal your body, mind and spirit, repair its organs and contribute to a longer, healthier, happier life.

Fasting benefits begin with the physical

First and foremost, benefits realized from fasting start in the physical realm. All other beneficial shifts – emotional, mental and spiritual – are well documented and piggyback off the physical changes. As your fast continues, you may notice additional benefits and positive effects not mentioned here.

Detoxification

"Fasting is an effective and safe method of detoxifying the body; a technique that wise men have used for centuries to heal the sick. Fast regularly and help the body heal itself and stay well. Give all of your organs a rest. Fasting can help reverse the aging process, and if we use it correctly, we will live longer, happier lives." –James Balch, M.D. *Prescription for Natural Healing.*

Detoxification is all about nourishing, resting and cleaning your body from its inside out. As soon as within 24-hours, your body begins to dramatically detoxify and you can actually *feel* changes beginning to occur. Your body is burning not only the natural toxins that occur in various foods and drinks, but the myriad of environmental poisons that irradiate and attack you on an aggressive, daily basis.

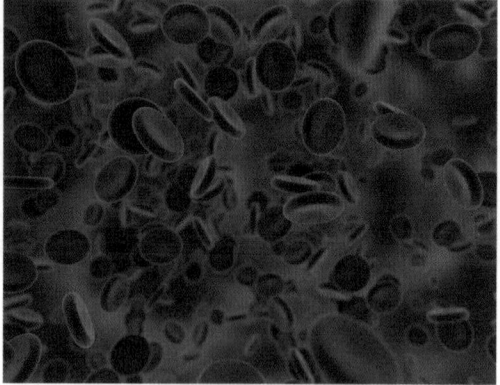

During your fast, your liver, kidneys, intestines and skin is stimulated to eliminate the accumulated poisons, a process that addresses *cells* - the smallest units of human life. Your body begins to rapidly eliminate digestive residues and the dead, dying and diseased cells that have not been excreted through normal detoxification. Everything, except vital tissue, will become eliminated; unwanted fatty tissue, the hard mucus coating of the intestinal wall, trans-fatty acids, deposits in the microscopic transports between your brain and the rest of your body, excess cholesterol and mucus from sinuses and your lungs.

Stress causes your body to release stress hormones into your system. In normal amounts, they can help you win a race or handle a 'fight or flight' situation, etc. But in large amounts, an over abundance of stress hormones create poisons that slow down the liver's normal detoxification process.

Physical healing

"A little starvation can really do more for the average sick man than can the best medicines and the best doctors. I do not mean a restricted diet; I mean total abstinence from food. I speak from experience; starvation has been my cold and fever doctor for 15 years, and has accomplished a cure in all instances." –Mark Twain (1835-1910).

Have you ever wondered why, when you're sick with a cold, the flu or other illness that you lose your appetite? It is because your body is initiating an 'involuntary fast.' It is slowing things down, dropping temperatures, diverting maintenance resources to healing, burning poisons and toxins and creating proteins, hormones and enzymes devoted to physical healing. When you purposely fast, you are *consciously* forcing the natural healing processes to occur.

Fasting has been proven or attributed in many situations to be a beneficial (if not the *only*) solution for Alzheimer's, arthritis, asthma, autoimmune disease, cases of paralysis, chronic fatigue, colitis, Crohn's disease, dementia, diverticulitis, eczema, some epileptic seizures, hypertension, irritable bowels, lupus, mental illness, neuralgia, neuritis, neuroses, pancreatitis, reducing cholesterol, rosacea, spastic colon, type II diabetes and many, many other conditions.

Spiritual benefits

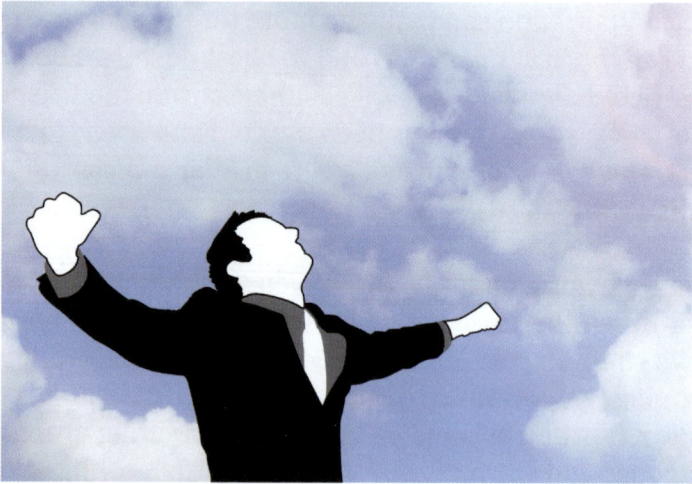

"If a person makes fasting part of her or his life, s/he'll experience a heightened spiritual awareness. By taking a long fast or two, and then fasting one day a week, s/he'll gradually find a growing peace and personal integration. America badly needs to go on a diet. It should do something drastic about excessive, unattractive, life-threatening fat. It should get rid of it in the quickest possible way, and this is by fasting." –Allan Cott, M.D. *Fasting: The Ultimate Diet.*

For centuries men and women from virtually every religious persuasion have partaken in fasts for simply spiritual growth, renewal and healing. It was one, dramatic way for them to become closer to their God.

Fasting is a humbling, contrite activity. It requires not only a certain mental fortitude to begin and continue, but a tremendous amount of personal sacrifice, will power and *surrender,* too.

Usually, as a normal human being you can actually *feel* when you are soul-sick or devoid of spiritual well being. There's no pep in your steps. Your shoulders slump, your gait slows as if burdened with the cares of the world and your heart becomes heavy and wearisome. You are 'poor in spirit.'

When you recognize your spiritual weaknesses, acknowledge and submit yourself to a higher power, you are surrendering *your* will. This is not an easy thing to do – in any century. And fasting helps you reach that peaceful plateau.

> **Tip**: Consider including prayer and meditation as part of you taking advantage of the full, spiritual spectrum of fasting.

Fasting helps you to understand deeper spiritual concerns. It helps to focus your normally diverted attention on to matters of the soul, your *being*. It brings alive in you the ability to better exercise self-control in your life. Fasting liberates you from the slavery to your appetite and frees you to focus on more meaningful things.

Mental and emotional benefits

One of the remarkable and proven benefits derived from fasting is the overall sense of rejuvenation and feeling of increased or extended life expectancy. Because of the improved immune system and increased hormone production, Human Growth Hormones and anti-aging hormones are produced and distributed more efficiently.

As the fasting continues, your mental awareness increases dramatically and your 'brain fog' dissipates. Most everyone who fasts boasts of no hunger and more energy than normal. The more your body detoxifies itself, the clearer you will be able to 'think.' Since digesting a meal requires a tremendous amount of nervous and blood energies, when not being used during fasting, those same energies are directed more towards mental activity and healing.

You will find that your mental and physical senses are heightened. You will experience, as the fasting duration progresses, increased feelings of euphoria and emotional stability. Fasting will awaken your creativity and intuitive senses.

"Life is slow suicide. Nine humans in ten are suicides." - "To lengthen thy life, lessen thy meals." - "The best of all medicines are rest and fasting."—Benjamin Franklin, LL.D. (1706-1790).

Fasting for weight loss

One of the primary reasons people participate in a fast is to lose weight and weight loss during a fast happens extremely quickly. As your body sheds the poisons, dead and dying cells, excess water and turns the fat into energy, it is not uncommon to lose two to three pounds in the first 72 hours and upwards of a pound per day for as long as you continue your fast. And the more obese you are, the more dramatic the weight losses.

The human body is valued at 3,500 calories per pound of fat. The amount of calories required, as energy to *lose* that pound of fat is 3,500. It varies between individuals based on health, height, overall weight and metabolism and activity levels. But the average adult burns anywhere between 1,800 and 3,500 calories a day.

As your metabolism slows towards the waning days of your fast, of course the energy requirement decreases and less weight is lost. But if you balance the slowed metabolism with increased –

but safe and reasonable exercise – your weight loss can remain steady and be significant.

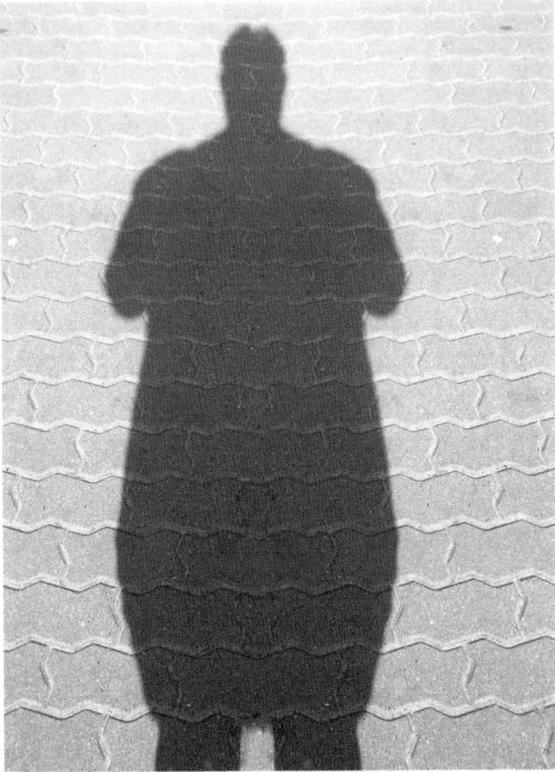

Juice Fasting and Detoxification

"The ideal technique for successful fasting is the use of fresh, raw fruit and vegetable juices. On such a diet, the full spectrum of nutrients is supplied in an easily assimilated form, so the digestive tract is able to remain essentially at rest. It is only through the combined use of both cleansing processes, and a very good diet, that one will be able to reach her or his maximal level of physical health and an unclouded consciousness." -- Rudolph Ballentine, M.D. *Diet & Nutrition.*

What is a juice fast?

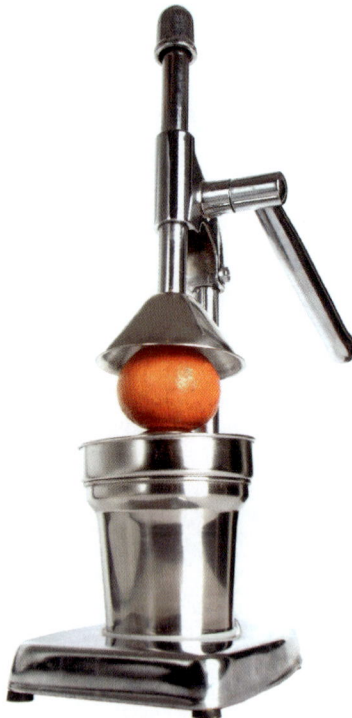

Our bodies were designed to thrive on raw – not cooked - vegetables. Juice fasting is as it says: a one day to five week detoxification fast or diet where water, vegetable and fruit juices replace solid or 'chewing' food. It is generally accepted that a 10-day water fast equals a 30-day juice fast.

It is not necessarily a safe idea to undertake a liquid-protein fast. Unless you are extremely obese, this diet should *only* be undertaken with the strict guidance and monitoring of your physician.

Benefits of juice fasts

As with regular water only fasting, juice fasts offer similar benefits with fewer side effects:

> Loss of weight
> Lower blood pressure
> Delays the onset of age-related diseases such as Alzheimer's and diabetes
> Has been linked to the prevention of heart disease
> Cleanses the poisonous toxins from your body
> Physically repairs your body
> Improved skin tone
> Eliminates or reduces allergy symptoms
> Gives you mental clarity
> Facilitates restful sleep
> Actually contributes to a longer life

What side effects can you experience?

As in all fasts, there may be some temporary side effects of a juice fast. These can commonly include headaches, hunger, hypoglycemia, changed in sleep patterns and increased dreaming, constipation or diarrhea (which can lead to loss of electrolytes and dehydration), dizziness or light-headedness, tiredness, acne and other skin eruptions, aches and pains, increased body odor, and bad breath. Acidic juices such as tomatoes, grapefruits and other citrus fruits may cause stomach pain or minor discomfort from acidy effects on your digestive system.

More significant side effects can include fainting and dizziness, lowered blood pressure, heart arrhythmias, excessive weight loss, vomiting, and kidney issues. If these side effects happen or your symptoms get worse or new symptoms appear, you should discontinue fasting and immediately see a qualified healthcare professional.

Lengthy juice fasts can lead to protein, calcium and other nutrient deficiencies.

Juice fasting recommendations

Keep in mind that the preparation time, techniques, fasting times and durations as well as the termination of your fast is very similar to water-only fasting. Remember that it is wise to seek the guidance of your doctor or healthcare professional if you decide to undertake a juice fast.

Generally speaking, you can do a juice fast for a longer period if time, as well as more frequently. Other than solid foods, you are taking in nourishment – calories, nutrients, vitamins and essential minerals.

Drink fresh juice. They have no additives such as flavorings (huh?), coloring, additional sugars and salts or other ingredients you would find in bottled and canned juices. Remember, you're *detoxing*! And remember to check with the juice bar baristas when drinking juice out. They will tell you if their juice blends are packaged, frozen or fresh.

Another consideration to keep in mind when drinking grapefruit, Pomelos and Seville oranges, as well as some other citrus juices is that they may *seriously* interact with some types of prescription medications you may be taking. The natural chemicals in grapefruits interfere with your body's enzymes that metabolize various medications through your digestive system. Consequently, the medicine stays in your body, which can increase the potency to potentially dangerous and unpredictable levels. Here are just a few examples of prescription medication-grapefruit interactions:

buspirone
amiodarone
Simvastatin, lovastatin, atorvastatin
saquinavir, indinavir
sertraline
ebastine
felodipine, nifedipine
triaxzolam, carbamazepine, diaxzepam, midazolam
carbamaxzepine
nifedipine, nimodipine
nisoldpine
methadone
saquinavir
cyclosporine, tacrolimus, sirolimus

This is by no means an exhaustive list, so again, please verify the possible interactions you may experience with your medical professional.

How much juice should you drink?

If you think about juice as being your entire food for the day, a gallon of juice would not be too much. It is an individual choice and based on your goals. One good rule-of-thumb would be to drink one, 8-12 ounce glass of juice every one-and-a-half hour. This will keep you on top of your hunger pangs and satisfy your bodily requirements for the goal you have in mind. But your fluid intake will most likely vary from one day to the next. Like eating chewable, solid food however, don't 'drink' to satisfy your mood or make you emotionally feel better.

Terminating a juice fast

Ending a juice fast is similar to terminating a water-only fast. Except that you don't need to make the transition to eating by drinking some vegetable or fruit juices – you're already there.

The day the fast ends, start by eating some simple fruits and vegetables. Don't eat a lot and don't eat too fast. Your digestive system will probably already be flushed, but it's been almost completely idle and at rest throughout your fast, so it just needs to readjust to solid foods. Wait for an hour or so and then eat again. Do this again throughout the first day. Simple fruits such as apples and vegetables such as a simple salad will slowly kick-start your digestive metabolism.

On day two, begin with an expanded selection of fruit – a banana, a grapefruit (if your medications allow it) or a peach. For lunch, have an 8-12 ounce bowl of soup and for dinner, another vegetable (and fruit) salad. Dry, 100% whole-wheat toast with any of the meals is also a great addition. And be sure to keep up your water-hydration throughout the day – 64-96 ounces of distilled or purified water.

As time goes on, you can slowly reenter the land of the 'chewing.' For the first three-to-five days, avoid heavier cooked foods until you are convinced that your body is ready.

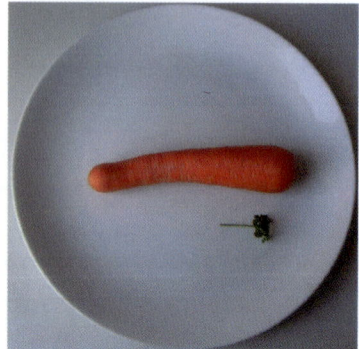

Your Common Sense Guide to Fasting - Successful 24-hour, 3-day, and Multi-week Fasts

For over 7,000 years and quite possibly longer, fasting has been a part of the human experience. The early proponents lived in a *culture* of fasting; it went on all the time somewhere and in someone around them. So, they knew and were aware of the effects, limitations, benefits and dangers of fasting. As the practice has diminished over the centuries, so has the knowledge of not only the benefits and encumbrances, but the techniques as well. Who should and shouldn't fast? How long should you fast and when should you quit fasting? Should you undertake a dry fast, water-only fast or a juice fast? And what can you expect to happen during a fast?

Individuals who should not fast

> Nursing mothers
> Anorexic or Bulimic individuals
> Pregnant, diabetic women
> Anyone with severe anemia
> Individuals who are too old that their body chemistry can no longer support safe fasting
> Some individuals who have a rare, genetic fatty acid deficiency which prevents proper ketosis from occurring
> Those with porphyria

Those who should fast under the close supervision of a Doctor or Medical Practitioner

Women who are pregnant
Young children and infants
Individuals with diminished kidney function
Those with Type I diabetes
Someone who might have a serious disease
Individuals who may have a significant fear of fasting but
wish to do so anyway
Individuals using prescriptions should not fast longer
than three days without supervision
Patients who have cancer, a chronic degenerative or
tuberculosis

How long and how often should you fast?

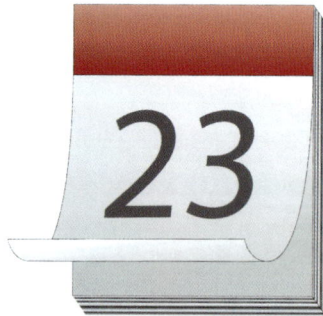

Traditionally, fasts are one, 3, 10 30 and even up to 50 days long.
But there is no magic number. It is up to you and your individual
health needs, goals and mindset. Keep in mind though, that all
things being equal, longer fasts should definitely be carried out
under the supervision of a doctor or other healthcare
professional. As your body changes through detoxification it is
wise to monitor everything that's going on to avoid the
unnecessary risks and dangerous side effects you might
experience.

   Tip: Remain flexible. Avoid disappointment if your body
   is signaling you to terminate your fast early. And if you

are doing very well during your fast and desire to
continue, don't feel like you have to quit just because
you've reached or exceeded a predetermined milestone.

A one-day fast is a great place to start if you're new to fasting.
And 72-hours is generally easy for most people. You can use that
experience to learn exactly what *your* body is going to
experience during a fast, and to help you prepare for longer
periods of fasting.

Three-day fasts fit well into most of our busy schedules and are
an optimum 'weekend' fast. As with a one-day fast, it's fairly easy
to commit to 72 hours.

For one- and three-day fasts, it is a good idea to allow for a
preparation day ahead of the fast and a transition day following
the period of fasting. This gives you a period of time to mentally
prepare to fast as well as some time when fasting's over to
resume normal (or better) eating habits.

For the longer fasting periods, two, three, four weeks or more,
the preparation time and the terminal transition period should
be extended appropriately. It is not uncommon for both to be
equal to half of the total number of fasting days. So, for a seven-
day fast, roughly three days would be devoted to preparation
and transition time. For a 30-day fast, 15 days before and after
would be normal. Assuming you are not going to immediately
terminate your fast and jump right in to junk food, this transition
period becomes essential.

It is also important to determine how often you should fast. In
between fasting times, your body needs periods of time to
rebuild its nutritional reserves. For long fasts, one fast a year
would be about right. One to two medium fasting periods of 10-
14 days per year are also recommended. For maintenance and
detoxification fasts, one day a week or three days a month
should suffice.

Finally, when deciding how long and how often to fast, consider your goals as well as your lifestyle and commitments. The longer the fasting period, the greater the commitment of not only you, but your family members and friends will be, too.

Step-by-Step Fasting for Better Health – How to Fast and What to Expect

"I fast for greater physical and mental efficiency." --Plato (428-348 B.C.)

In the previous few chapters I've covered a lot of ground regarding the *why's* of fasting - what is it, its benefits and disadvantages, side-effects, types, duration and frequency of fasts. Now it's time to get started and with the actual *how's*. I've drawn from my own personal experiences as well as the myriad of people I've coached and interviewed before, during and after their fasts. Oh, and I'll share some insight into what you might expect, too.

Prepare, prepare, prepare

Mental preparation

Fasting, whether it's a 24-hour or a 5-week fast requires some preparation. In actuality, getting started on a fast is almost the hardest part. Your mind is going to do *everything* to convince you not to deprive *its* body of food and nourishment. The more prepared you are, the easier the transition to the fast will be.

First, you need to get your mind around the idea. A lot of self-talk goes a long way, here. It is proven that if you talk 'out-loud' to yourself in positive sentences, your psyche will believe it. Thoughts help, but don't work in the same way. You have to 'hear' it.

So, ridiculous as it may seem, give yourself some positive 'pep talks.' Look into the mirror if it helps. 'It's going to be a *great* three-day fast and *I can do it!*' 'I am going to look and feel *so good* after just two weeks of a juice fast. I can hardly wait!'

Stick Post-it notes in places you'll see them. Post them in the car, on the bathroom mirror, on the refrigerator door or on the lampshade beside your bed. 'I will embrace the detoxification.' 'I am looking forward to fasting.' 'This fast will be easy.' Whatever you need to read that will get you into the mental *groove*.

Think of fasting as a vacation away from your normal living patterns. You're going on a fasting trip *and* looking forward to it as an adventure.

While fasting is and of itself a personal trek, it is wise to elicit the encouragement of your family and friends. Don't get into negative discussions with the naysayers, but do surround yourself with those who will give you not only encouragement to start, but also ongoing affirmations to continue and succeed.

> **Tip**: If you are initiating a weight loss fast, then another trick is to take and hang a photo of your current self in a prominent place for you to see (or put it in your wallet, if you'd rather not have it made public). This becomes not only a motivator, but the 'before' picture of your vacation.

Spiritual preparation

If you have spiritual tendencies and believe in a higher power, here is a good place for prayer and spiritual preparation. Your body is weak; your mind may be willing but quite often your spirituality is what gives you the edge.

Logistics

Believe it or not, fasting isn't just something as simple as saying, 'I'm going to fast for a week,' then fast for seven days, then stop and return to your normal life. It takes preparation; follow-through and a transition back to a healthy normal diet.

The logistics of fasting are as important to the arrangements as the mental and spiritual preparations. So, clean out your refrigerator. According to how long your fast is, the food in there will either (1) spoil or (2) prevent your start or (3) tempt you to failure. Put it in the freezer. Give it to family or friends, but remove it from sight. It's akin to leaving a dog-bone in front of your pet's nose and telling him "*no!*"

Second, clear your schedule if you're planning a short, one to three-day fast or make arrangements to accommodate your activities if it will be longer. If you will be fasting over a weekend, don't plan on Saturday girl's night out (unless you have tremendous self-discipline.) If you will be fasting for two or three weeks or more keep in mind the tamale vendor at work, coffee and Danish with Mom on Thursdays, Sunday potlucks after church and Friday night dates. Even a movie out becomes a temptation. The longer the fast, the more of your life you'll have to rearrange in order to accommodate it. And by all means, when you are out or have an activity come up that involves food that you can't work around, seek the support of someone else in attendance. Most of your activities include family and friends, *so utilize them!*

Third, if you are planning to fast for 10-days or more, it is extremely prudent to share your plans with someone close to you who can help 'keep an eye out.' Even more imperative than telling a close friend or family member is notifying your doctor or other healthcare professional of your intentions. Because of your own health situation, there may be some tests he or she may want to undertake or some other considerations that need to be discussed or addressed before you embark on such a serious venture.

Prior to launch day you should begin to scale back on your meal portions. Not only will this strengthen your mindset, but also it will help your body begin to function differently; as if it realizes energy supplies are becoming scarce or non-existent. It is a good idea to wean yourself of caffeine and sugar, as well.

The day before your fast begins, eat several small meals about every two hours. Drink plenty of water and the night before your fast begins, eat only a light dinner. Make sure it has a high, carbohydrate content. Eat slowly, enjoy it and again, drink plenty of water. Resist the urge to have that 'last, big meal.'

Keep in mind that the more time you devote to the physical preparation for your fast, the easier it will be to make the transition from eating to fasting.

> **Tip**: If you are new to fasting, it is a good idea to observe a few 1- or 3-day fasts, going through the complete planning-fasting-termination lifecycle for practice in preparation for the longer, more difficult fasts.

Finally, if you are going to be fasting for 10 or more days, before you begin go out and buy some *ketone test strips* such as *Ketostix, Uriscan* and *Atkins.* You can get a bottle of 100 for $6-$12 from any pharmacy. Daily, during your fast, you will dip the strip's padded end into a fresh urine specimen. Almost immediately it will change color to indicate the level of ketone bodies detected. Based on the color, a urine value of 0 (negative) through 4+ (severe) indicates the level of *ketonuria* and acidosis. The higher your urine value determines whether or not you may be fasting safely or should immediately contact your healthcare provider and terminate your fast.

Additionally, you may want to purchase either distilled or purified water or a water filtering system, such as Brita, Pūr, or other cleansing filters. I prefer these options to tap water because of the toxins inherent in potable municipal water systems. After all, you *are* detoxing environmental poisons, too.

The fast is on!

Congratulations, you've begun! But today will be a difficult day. If you are undertaking a water-only fast, it will be even *more* difficult.

The first three days

Your cycle of eating and digestion has changed, and right off the bat you are going to notice that your body is beginning to revolt. It wants food. Based on when your previous afternoon or evening's light meal was eaten and what time you normally eat breakfast, you're already roughly 12- to 20-hours into your fast; your body will be screaming, "Hey, I'm getting hungry, here!" Get out of bed, brush your teeth and drink your first glass of water.

It is important while fasting to drink a significant amount of distilled or purified water so your body doesn't confuse thirst with hunger. A good, daily amount is to drink 64 to 96 ounces (eight to twelve, 8-oz glasses throughout the day.) This is going to keep you from becoming dehydrated and at the same time, help your body flush out the toxins and poisonous residue. Be careful not to over-hydrate or hydrate too quickly. You could inadvertently flush out important electrolytes too quickly. The modern rule-of-thumb for hydration is, 'drink as your thirst dictates.'

During the first three fasting days, your body wants to signal that it is hungry. And signal it will. And it will signal louder until you enter the physical stage of ketosis between 48 and 72 hours. Water helps ward off those hunger pangs, but will not eliminate them entirely. This is where the mental and spiritual changes begin to happen. In order to ignore these signals, you'll need to focus on other things. Think about other stuff. Concentrate. Pray.

Meditate. And *man up or woman up*, as they say to ignore or at least tolerate the internal screaming.

Two things that have been shown to alleviate the hunger pangs are psyllium bulk and silymarin tablets. They also aid in cleansing the body and especially the liver. Take one teaspoon of psyllium and mix it with some lukewarm distilled water. It will take on the consistency of Jell-O. It hastens the colon's toxin eliminations and in most people, will help eliminate dizziness and headaches. If you want to control your bad breath, alfalfa tablets work well. Take two tablets 3-4 times each day.

It is very important for you to continue to take all of your prescribed medications during your fast. You and your doctor may find a diminished need for some (such as for hypertension) but continue taking them unless otherwise directed by your physician.

The first three days are not fun and because they are so difficult, it is one of the main reasons many people terminate their fasts early. But if you can drive on through the discomfort, after day three you'll begin to realize remarkable changes.

If you are a heavy caffeine drinker, you may experience some headaches during these first few days. You will also notice that you may become tired and weaker than normal. Your metabolism is slowing down and conserving energy, waiting to be fed.

It is a good idea to exercise to help the toxins dissipate in your sweat. Don't just lie around. But don't exercise too strenuously, either, or you will deplete your body's electrolytes too quickly. Aggressive exercise raises the body temperature and causes you to sweat more aggressively, and thereby throw off those electrolytes. Most people have about a 30-day store of

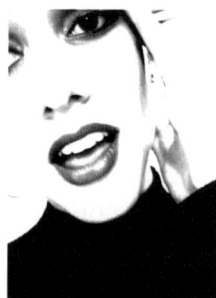

electrolytes as long as they are not particularly deficient in any of them.

When you stand, rise slowly and cautiously so you don't experience a faint.

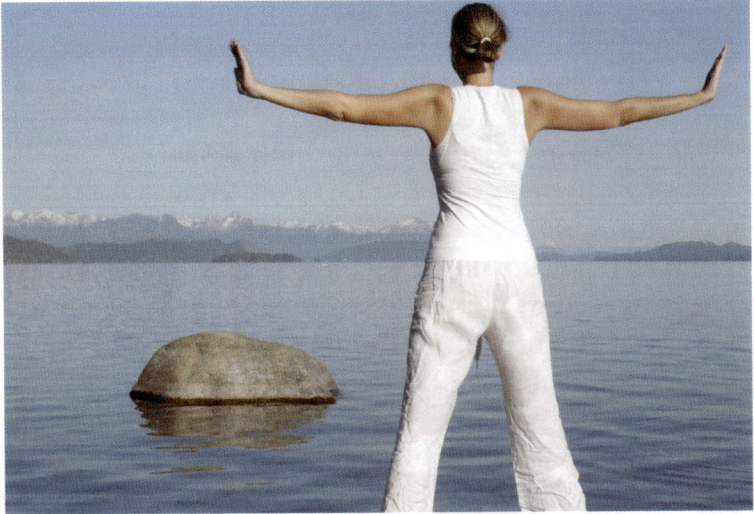

If this is your first fast, your detox symptoms will most likely be more significant than if you fast regularly. You've got a lot of junk inside your body that needs to come out. A few things you will notice is that your breath will begin to have an unpleasant smell and your body odor will increase. Your body will begin and continue to release poisons through your breathing (lungs), skin, urine and stool. You may experience diarrhea or constipation during this time, as well. Don't be overly concerned; these are normal side effects of fasting. They will surely dissipate.

You will also probably notice that your weight loss has begun and you've lost a pound or two at the start. Right now, your body is still burning up the food remaining in your stomach and colon and the by-products are getting flushed out.

The list of side effects for these first three days is by no means exhaustive. Everyone will generally experience common effects and you may experience more and different ones. You may also be one of the lucky ones who fast with few side effects to speak of. And as you fast more frequently, your body has already gone through its first detoxification, so subsequent fasts will not be as physically demanding as the first.

Days four and on to completion

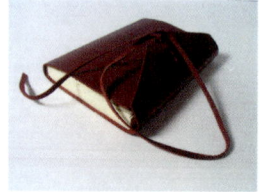

Tip: Now would be a good time to start keeping a fasting journal. This will help you not only in your present fast, but in future fasts, as well. Keep track of everything you notice; changes, weight loss, side effects, increased mental awareness and spiritual changes. By the end of your fast, you will be amazed at how your health has improved and your overall well being.

By day four, you should be in ketosis. Your body is now breaking down its fast stores for fuel. From here on out, it actually gets easier. One significant way to tell if you are in ketosis is that you may experience the odor of acetone in your breath and your tongue may become white-coated as toxins are pouring out from your lungs. Industrial acetone is the solvent used in some paints and fingernail polish remover, so you should be familiar with the odor. Again, don't be overly alarmed, it will go away, too.

Now is the day you start testing your urine with the ketone strips. Once a day is sufficient, but keep an eye on the readings. Notify your doctor if it rises significantly.

Keep up with your water intake. This cannot be understated. You will experience many detoxification side effects and it is important to keep the fluid coming. One pound of human flesh has a 3,500-calorie value. Water has no calories or nutritional value. So from here on out, your body has *no choice* but to turn to its internal fat stores to create energy.

Humans burn *on average* from 1,800 to about 3,500 calories per day. This, of course, depends on your age, general health, activity levels, heart rate and other factors. At 3,500 calories per pound of flesh, you'll need to burn 3,500 calories through normal and increased activity to lose that pound. Here is where your journal can come in handy. Write down and monitor your activities to keep track of the calories spent and the associated weight loss. You may notice a two to three pound per day loss during the first three days, due to passing a significant amount of sodium and water. In the latter stages (days 4+) your weight loss may drop down to only ½ a pound a day.

For several days you may notice increased – then diminished – detoxification side effects. You will be detoxifying from every orifice and organ, including your skin. Do not be alarmed if you experience increased pimples, acne or even boils. The poison is being pushed out through your skin. As your body becomes cleansed, these effects will go away.

One of the problems I've found during longer, 10+ days of fasting is *boredom.* We are social creatures and sharing meals with family, friends and co-workers is something we like to do. We also enjoy eating. People devote anywhere from two to three hours a day or more to just *eating.* It's no wonder that boredom will set in because now you've got to find something else to do during what would normally be mealtime or social eating. Remember though, not to put yourself into unnecessary situations where failure becomes a possibility.

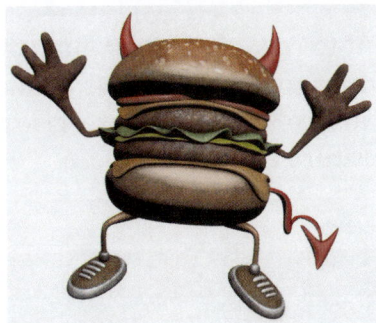

During these advanced fasting days, you will find that your mental acuity is increasing. Your thoughts will be quicker, fuller, more focused. Your memory becomes keener. This is a *noticeable* change.

It's over – terminating your fast

Congratulations! You've just completed your fast. It's time to return to the land of the eating.

The first thing to remember is that when you resume eating again begin lightly and gradually. This is especially true for longer fasts. Your digestive system has been at virtually a complete standstill for 10+ days. So don't rush out and grab that extra large hamburger funny meal.

Steamed or raw vegetables are best for terminating a fast, most experts agree. After a lengthier fast of 7+ days or more, your stomach will be smaller, so it's important to eat lighter. And it is important to stop eating *before* you feel full. Try to avoid starchy foods like white bread, potatoes, white rice or pastas for a week or more, as well as meats, fats, oils or dairy products. Reintroduce them in small amounts. 100% whole wheat bread and wild rice is ok.

Keep your hydration up, too. During the day drink as much purified or distilled water, as you like, trying to get in those 64-96 ounces.

Exercise is important to resume as well. But start slowly as you re-adjust your activities to pre-fast levels. Your metabolism will return to a new normal, so don't over exercise and thereby cause unnecessary temperature elevations.

Your first few meals

The first meals you eat following any fast are just as important whether you fasted for three days or four weeks. Here are some recommendations:

Your first meal should be limited to five or six whole, medium tomatoes, peeled, chopped and steamed. When they're cool, you can eat as many of them as you like.

Your first breakfast should consist of a small salad of fresh grated cabbage and carrots. ½ of an orange squeezed over the salad makes an excellent natural dressing. Before you eat though, drink two 8-oz glasses of water with ½ of a lemon juice squeezed in. Add a little salt so that the drink tastes both salty and lemony. Drink these and after a bit, eat your breakfast. The lemon and salt-water will help awaken your digestive system and cause it to flush with a strong bowel movement, removing any remaining poisons.

For lunch, you can again have the steamed tomatoes with some greens added in. Also, one or two slices of 100% whole-wheat toast (completely dry) may be eaten. This may help with any feelings of nausea you may experience.

For dinner, have first a salad of chopped celery and grated carrots and cabbage. Add the ½ freshly squeezed orange juice. Then two steamed vegetables. Eat one, which comes from the greens family and one of carrots, celery, okra, squash, or string

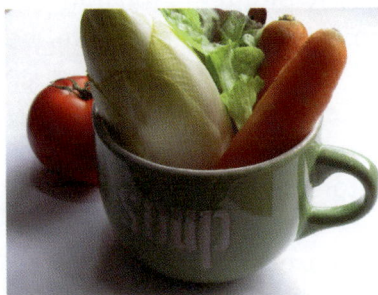

beans. You may also have the one or two slices of 100% whole-wheat toast (completely dry).

On the following day breakfast will consist of a dish of any fruit. Add two tablespoons of raw wheat germ and sweeten it with no more than one tablespoonful of honey.

For lunch you can have a small salad of fresh chopped celery, grated cabbage and carrots. With the orange dressing and one to two pieces of the dry, whole-wheat toast (so dry that you can crumble it up).

Finally, for dinner you may have a lettuce, watercress, tomato and parsley salad and two steamed vegetables.

Change your eating lifestyle

Now is a great time to change your eating habits. If you are overweight or obese, learn *now* about a proper diet and portion control. It makes little sense to struggle through even a three day fast, much less 10+ days and go right back to your old, poor eating habits. You've just won the battle of mind over body and you should be rejuvenated and strengthened to carry this forward for a healthier life.

This is one area where the mental and spiritual benefits can follow you well after your fast is over. Now is also the time to begin planning your next fasting experience, whether it's a short fast a week away or a longer fast in six months.

Claim and direct your newly found mental and spiritual awakening towards gaining and keeping discipline in your life.

I hope *The Complete Fasting Guide To Miraculous Health And Well-Being* has been a blessing to you. Not just a big gob of information, but also a starting point to learn about and actually begin a fast – *and succeed.* Remember to do your due diligence by reading and studying more about fasting. Join a fasting group or forum and ask questions. Rely on your medical care practitioner or doctor for insight and support.

Take what you've learned and apply it to the real world of fasting. Plan it, do it and enjoy all of the benefits that are sure to come your way. You will be amazed and surprised at the results.

Here's to a *better you* through safe fasting!

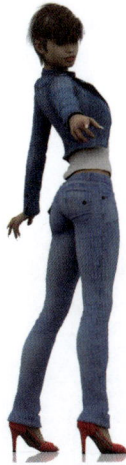

The Recipes - Juice Fasting and Detoxification Recipes

Here you will find 40+ delicious recipes that will serve you during your juice fast. There are purees, soups and blended salads. As you make the transition from fasting back to eating again, many of the recipes can be made to eat instead of drink and guide you through that transition. As your healthy lifestyle continues, these recipes can become part of your eating and drinking habits due to their slimming and detox effects on your body and organs.

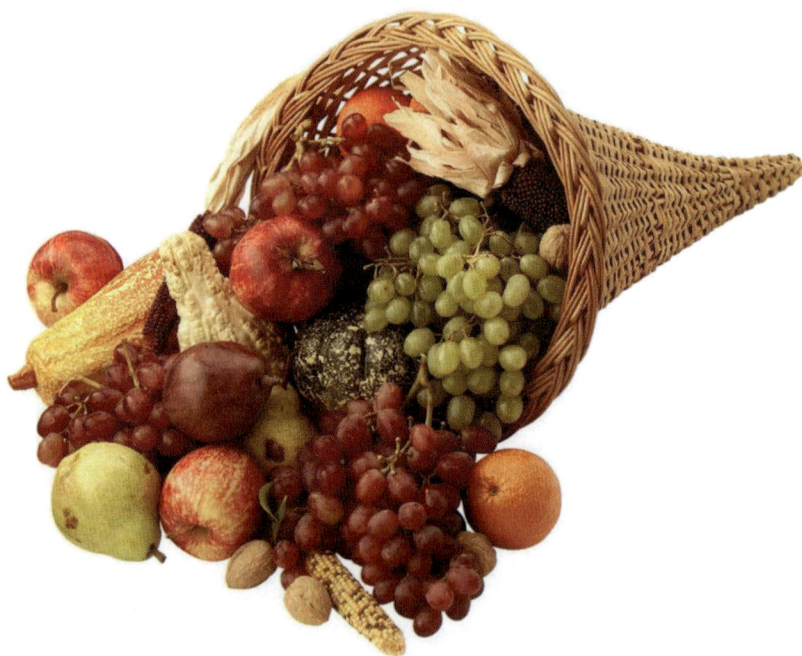

D

uring liquid fasting and detoxification dieting, it is essential to feed your metabolism with as much nutrient energy as you can. Depending on your health needs and the type of detox fast or diet you are on, vegetables and fruit juices as well as some liquid-protein drinks all do the work of cleansing your body, resting your digestive system and eliminating toxins from your body.

In this section of the book, you will find soups, drinks and blended salads that are both tasty and varied to keep boredom during a lengthy fast or diet to a minimum. These recipes are all flexible in their ingredients so be creative; mix them to fit your own detoxification plan. If you are on a liquid-only fast, then most of the recipes can be blended to make a delicious drink, some by adding water, juices or milks made from allowed foods. If you are on a 'chewing' detox diet, then of course you can mix and match foods according to your own detox plan.

Here is a list of the various food groups that contribute well to juice and detoxification fasts and diets.

Vegetables: fresh broccoli, onions, cauliflower, garlic, dark leafy greens such as collard greens, swish chard and kale, artichokes, kelp, wakame, beets, bell peppers, eggplants, nori sheets and potatoes. Avoid canned vegetables. They are high in sodium and preservatives.

Fruits: fresh or frozen (avoid canned), unsweetened, natural fruit juices, dried fruit such as raisins, dates and cranberries.

Grains and starches: brown rice, millet, wild rice, quinoa, oats, buckwheat, amaranth.

Oils: hemp, flax, chia, cold-pressed, extra-virgin olive, avocado, coconut and almond oils.

Condiments: Bragg's Liquid Aminos, miso, apple cider vinegar, lemons and limes, dried fresh herbs and spices, cacao nibs and power, carob powder, mustard and sea salt.

Sweeteners: black strap molasses, raw honey, stevia, real maple syrup, erythritol, brown rice syrup.

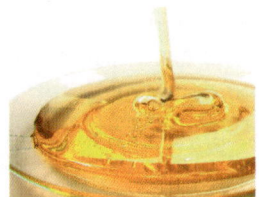

Beans and legumes: lentils, adzuki beans, split yellow and green peas.

Animal proteins (if required for safe and healthy detox): wild game, lamb, organic chicken and turkey, Alaskan salmon, wild, cold-water fish.

Beverages: herbal, ginger and green teas, lemon and lime water, mineral and seltzer water, unsweetened fresh fruit and vegetable juice, water, fresh coconut, hemp, rice and almond milks.

Nuts and seeds: raw and unsalted almonds, cashews, walnuts, coconuts, sunflower, sesame, chia and pumpkin seeds, hemp nuts and seeds, tahini, butters made from allowed ingredients.

It is important while fasting to drink a significant amount of distilled or purified water so your body doesn't confuse thirst with hunger. A good, daily amount is to drink 64 to 96 ounces (eight to twelve, 8-oz glasses throughout the day.) This is going to keep you from becoming dehydrated and at the same time, help your body flush out the toxins and poisonous residue. Be careful not to over-hydrate or hydrate too quickly. You could inadvertently flush out important electrolytes too quickly. The modern rule-of-thumb for hydration is, 'drink as your thirst dictates.'

> **Tip**: always carefully wash the fruits and vegetables going into a juice blend with filtered or distilled water. Remember that one of the purposes of fasting and detoxification is to eliminate many of the environmental poisons from our bodies. City water is often *rife* with these toxins.

It is recommended that you take in some sort of drink or liquid nourishment every 1-½ to 2 hours throughout the day to stay ahead of the hunger feelings. This keeps your

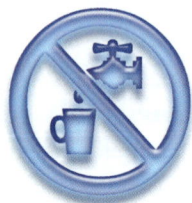

metabolism and energy levels up. Like eating chewable, solid food however, don't 'drink' to satisfy your mood or make you emotionally feel better.

Veggie Combo Detox Drink
1 serving

1/2 of a beetroot
2 or 3 sprigs of watercress
2 Swiss chard leaves
3 carrots
1 celery stalk
After you have completely washed the ingredients with distilled or filtered water, cut them up and blend them in a juicer.

Tart and Light
1 serving

1 cup red grapes
1-1/2 cups of chopped or diced fresh pineapple
1 red grapefruit
After you have washed the ingredients chop them up, blend them and

Pick-me-up Energy Drink
1 serving

1 organic, skins-on cucumber
1/2 of a beet
1/2 of a lemon
1/2 of a carrot
2 celery stalks
a handful of fresh parsley

Wash the ingredients water, cut them up and blend them in a juicer.

Kale is like *Superman*!
1 serving

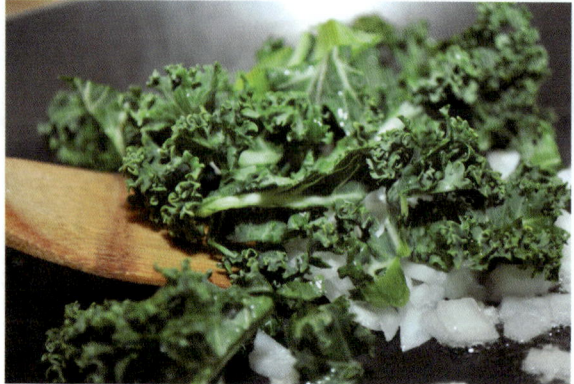

6 Kale Leaves
4 Celery Stalks
1 Cucumber
1/2 Lemon
1 piece of ginger
2 Green Apples

After you have completely washed the ingredients with distilled or filtered water, cut them up and blend them in a juicer.

Fruit Milkshake
1 serving

Besides being very tasteful, strawberries are one of nature's healthiest fruits. Strawberries are extremely rich in potassium. They have a lot of iron and vitamin C, so they can be used to treat anemia. Both strawberries and bilberries have high antioxidant properties, but they cannot compare to those of chokeberries. Chokeberries have one of the highest levels of antioxidants of all fruits and vegetables. Antioxidants stop cell destruction, thus can help cancer treatment.

1 ounce of strawberries
1 ounce of bilberries
1 ounce of chokeberries (aronia)

1 banana
1 avocado
4 ounces of soymilk

Blend the fruit to make paste, add to milk and shake altogether. If you prefer you can leave berries whole.

Stinging Nettle Hot Drink

This is one very tasteful dish composed with the purpose of introducing stinging nettle into regular culinary use. Stinging nettle is rich in nutrients perfect for detoxification. It helps excretion of toxins from the body and gives strength and energy. Stinging nettle is a traditional remedy for anemia, enlarged prostate, troubled digestion and respiratory system diseases.

3 ounces of stinging nettle leaves
3 ounces of soymilk
1 onion
1 garlic clove
Pinch of salt and pepper
2 tablespoons of olive oil

Cook the stinging nettle leaves in salted water for twenty minutes. Strain the leaves and cut through the mass or blend it for only few seconds to make paste. In another pan put chopped onion, garlic, and oil, and cook it for two-to-three minutes. Next, add the stinging nettle, and after two-to-three minutes add soymilk. Remove from the heat and serve while hot.

Marshmallow and Dandelion Tea
1 serving

The main purpose of marshmallow and dandelion tea is to help in kidney detoxification. Marshmallow is a well-known plant for its anti-inflammatory properties, while dandelion improves overall health of your body.

½ ounce of marshmallow root
½ ounce of dandelion leaves
1 teaspoon of honey
6 ounces of water

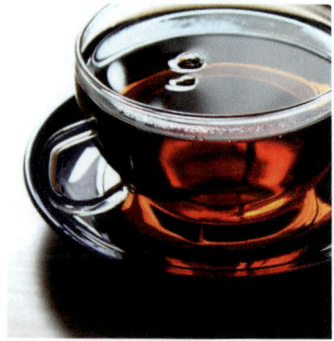

Boil the water for 1 minute, and then let it cool. Water must not be too hot because high temperature affects starch from marshmallow. After a while, when the water is lukewarm, pour it over the other ingredients. Let it rest for two-to-three hours, and then strain it. You can add a teaspoon or two of honey to improve the taste.

Everyday Bilberry Drink
1 serving

Bilberries are filled with vitamin C, organic acids, vitamin B and tannins. This fruit is used for fighting off various bacterial infections and fungal diseases. Knowing that boiling causes vitamin C loss, you should use bilberry fruit raw. Mixed with lemon juice and soymilk, bilberries make a real vitamin bomb, which can be consumed several times every day. Adding a bit of honey makes this beverage very tasteful. Feel free to drink as much as you like and don't worry about overdosing - bilberry fruit is used as preventive and remedy for both avitaminosis (any disease caused by chronic vitamin deficiencies) and hypovitaminosis (over-retention of fat-soluble vitamins in your body).

4 ounces of bilberry fruit
2 tablespoons of lemon juice

1 tablespoon of honey
5 ounces of soymilk

Blend the bilberries and mix with other ingredients.

Wheat Germ Drink
1 serving

Wheat germ is a powerful natural antioxidant and should make up part of almost every detox diet. It is rich in essential fatty acids, zinc, and magnesium. Mixed with fruit and yogurt, it makes one healthy, refreshing, and tasty drink.

1 handful of wheat germ
1 grated apple
1-2 teaspoons of brown sugar
7 ounces of unsweetened and unsalted yogurt drink or soymilk

Soak the wheat germ into the milk or yogurt for half an hour before mixing with apples and brown sugar.

Sport Mix
1 serving

Bananas are abundant with vitamins, minerals, trace elements, and have a very high nutritional value. Bananas are easy to digest and don't burden the stomach. Pumpkin seeds contain amino acids of high quality, while skim milk contains around 3 percent of protein. When you mixed all together you get a high-quality protein beverage, rich in fibers, and without simple carbs that can make you fat. This drink is especially recommended for athletes and for everyone who is under a lot of physical and mental stress.

2 bananas
2 tablespoons of pumpkin seeds
7 ounces of skim milk

Blend bananas and pumpkin seeds, and mix it together with the skim milk.

Beetroot Juice
1 serving

Beetroot is a food good for fighting cancer, anemia, bacterial infections, and some studies have shown that regular consuming of beetroot juice slows aging. It is very rich in iron, which works best with vitamin C. That is why this drink contains fruits such as oranges, lemon, pomegranate, and grapefruit. Mix it with brown sugar or honey and you will get one tasty and refreshing drink.

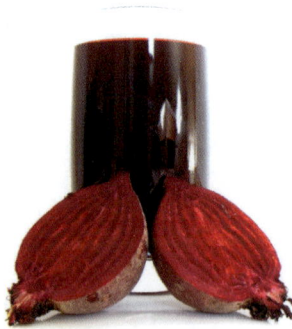

4 ounces of beetroot
1 orange
1 tablespoon of lemon juice
½ pomegranate
½ grapefruit
1 teaspoon of brown sugar or honey (optional)
4 ounces of water

Pour 4 ounces of water over blended beetroot and leave it in the refrigerator for 24 hours. After that you need to squeeze the mixture to get clear juice. Blend the rest of the ingredients and mix with the beetroot juice.

Energizing Orange Juice
1 serving

This is a protein-rich drink made of coconut powder, hazelnuts, and fresh orange juice. It is rich in vitamins such as vitamin C and vitamin E that protect the body from cancer and coronary disease. Proteins from coconut and hazelnuts have high quality profile of essential amino acids. Also, this drink is rich in essential fatty acids. High-energy value per serving is perfect for athletes and active persons, but those on fat-loss diet should use it sparingly.

8 ounces fresh orange juice
2 tablespoons coconut powder
2 tablespoons grounded hazelnuts
1 tablespoons honey or brown sugar

Put oranges through juicer or squeeze them to make 8 ounces of juice. Grind the hazelnuts and add them together with coconut powder and honey or brown sugar to the orange juice.

Oat Milkshake
1 serving

Oats are one of the most complete plants in terms of nutrients. Oats contains most of the vitamins and minerals essential for proper body functioning. When you combine oats with ribes, you get a drink that can help you fight kidney and liver disease, anemia, gout and high cholesterol. This drink helps whole body detoxification.

1 cup of ribes (currants or gooseberries)
2 tablespoons of oat germ
6 ounces of oat milk
1 tablespoon of honey

Ribes are often so tiny they do not have to be chopped or blended; just put everything altogether and mix.

Mint Ice Tea
1 serving

Use this drink when you need some rejuvenating refreshment. Lemon and orange juice will give you necessary vitamins, while mint will supply you with essential oils that gently act on your digestive system. This drink can sometimes help ease headaches, arrhythmia and nausea.

6 ounces of mint tea
3 ounces of fresh orange juice
2 tablespoons of lemon juice
1 tablespoon of honey

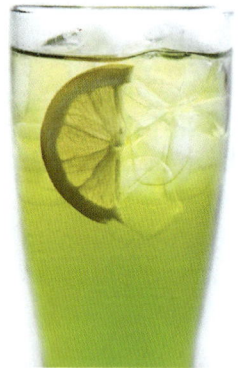

Pour boiling water over two teabags of mint tea (or two teaspoons). Strain after 10 minutes and put in refrigerator to cool. When you want to drink it, just mix it with fresh orange juice and lemon. Use honey as sweetener and add ice.

C-Bomb

1 serving

This drink is one very energizing drink, highly recommended for everyone on low-carb or detox diet. It is made of fruits that are rich in all essential vitamins and minerals. Every ingredient of this drink contains high amount of vitamin C. Only one serving contains around 1/3 of recommended daily amounts of vitamin C.

1 banana
5 ounces of fresh orange juice
5 ounces of beetroot nectar
1 lemon

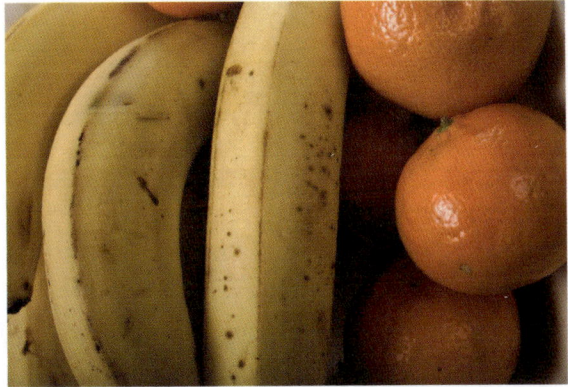

Blend one whole lemon (along with lemon peel) and one banana, and mix it with equal amounts of orange and beetroot juice.

Creamy Tomato Drink
1 serving

This drink is a must when on a detox diet. Tomatoes contain powerful antioxidant named lycopene, which fights free radicals responsible for cancer. Peppers contain more vitamin C than most of other vegetables, and vitamin C is also powerful antioxidant. Yogurt bacteria and spices such as pepper and ginger are a remedy for digestive troubles.

3 ounces of tomatoes
5 ounces of unsalted and unsweetened yogurt
2 bell peppers
Pinch of black pepper

Pinch of ginger
Pinch of rosemary
Half teaspoon of coriander

Peel tomatoes, squash them, and add to yogurt along with bell peppers and spices. Blend into a smoothie-drink.

Detox Power Drink
1 serving

This drink is designed to accelerate the body's detoxification processes. Black radish is probably the most powerful detox vegetable. It fights high cholesterol and fat. Black radish is powerful natural diuretic. It stimulates excretion of substances that are bad for body health. During that process, some minerals will excrete too. That is why this drink contains ingredients that can compensate mineral loss.

5 ounces of fresh black radish juice
2 tablespoons of apple vinegar
2 ounces of blended quince
1 ounce of blended Brazil nuts
1 tablespoon of honey

Blend pealed radishes, quinces, and Brazil nuts until mushy. Blend the mixture with other ingredients. If you feel that the drink is overly dense, add some purified water.

Garlic Soup
1 serving

During a detox diet the body suffers stress and physical effort, thus is subject to various infections. This soup is designed to raise the level of immunity. It is rich in vitamin C and other vitamins and minerals that will boost your immune system to fight bacteria and viruses. Hot and spicy properties of chili peppers and garlic are tempered with milk, or even better plain yogurt. Mixed altogether it makes one tasty soup suitable for everyday consumption.

2 tablespoons of chopped garlic
2 tablespoons of butter or olive oil
5 ounces of plain, non-fat yogurt or soymilk
2 ounces of tomato juice
2 small chili peppers
2 carrots

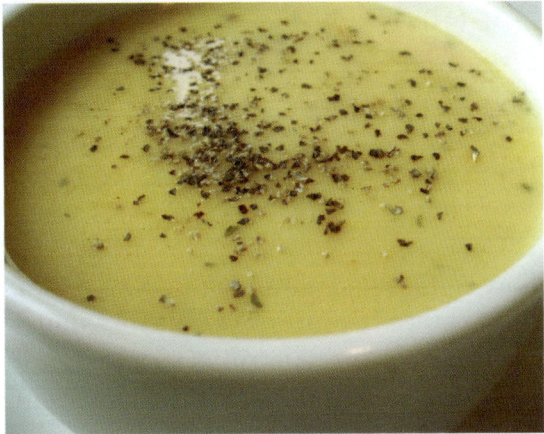

Sauté the garlic, peppers, and chopped carrots on oil for about three minutes. Than add tomato juice and yogurt. Wait until soup starts to boil and immediately move it from the heat. Let it cool a bit and consume it lukewarm. Strain the solid ingredients out or blend everything together in a blender.

Energizing Shitake Soup
1 serving

Whether you are fighting cancer or you just want to improve your overall health, this soup is excellent choice. All of the ingredients in this recipe are known as good antioxidants. Research conducted by Japanese scientists has shown that consuming shitake mushrooms helps tumor growth in 60 percent of cases. Lentil germ, soymilk, and parsley, all have high nutritional value, and combined with shitake mushrooms will make one highly energizing meal which will invigorate the whole body.

½ cup of shitake mushrooms
2 tablespoons of lentil germ
6 ounces of soymilk
Salt and pepper are optional

Add chopped mushrooms and germ to milk and heat it up to 40°C (103°F).

Kohlrabi Salad Blend
1 serving

Low calorie value and high vitamin and fiber value are the most important attributes of kohlrabi salad. Its antioxidant properties protect body from various sicknesses, including cancer. Kohlrabi salad is recommended for those with high blood pressure or hearth disease. It can be served as a salad or as a drink, depending on whether you chop or blend its ingredients.

1 cup of chopped kohlrabi
1 onion
1 tablespoon of cumin
1 tablespoon of flax seed
1 tablespoon of apple vinegar

Chop or blend the ingredients.

Healthy Brown Rice Salad
1 serving

In order to function properly, the body needs to be supplied with

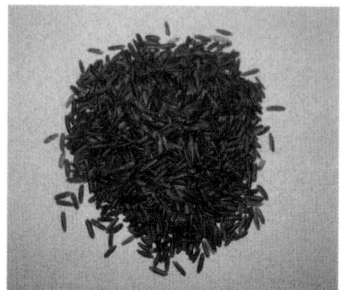

enough high-quality carbs. One of the healthiest sources of carbohydrates is brown rice. Combined with other ingredients, brown rice makes a tasty meal. It will give you feeling of being satisfied while providing you with a reasonable amount of calories.

1 cup of brown rice
1 small chili pepper
2 ounces of chopped black olives2-4 cloves of garlic

On the day before you plan to eat this meal you need to soak the rice into water and leave it there for 24 hours. After a day in water, rice needs to be strained. Chop peppers, olives and garlic, and add to rice.

Cauliflower Salad Blend
1 serving

Everyone who is on some fat-loss diet is looking for a meal that has high nutritional value and low calorie value. This recipe's main ingredient is cauliflower – plant that has those properties. It can be used in low-carb diets, because cauliflower has a lot of dietary fibers instead of simple carbs. Onion and spices are guarantee of taste.

5-7 ounces cauliflower
1 onion
1 teaspoon of parsley
1 tablespoon of apple vinegar
½ teaspoon of sea salt
½ teaspoon dill seeds
½ teaspoon sesame
½ teaspoon of coriander powder
½ teaspoon basil
1-3 ounces of yogurt or cabbage cheese

Chop cauliflower altogether with its leaves and boil it for 15 minutes. Strain it and mix with other ingredients. Serve cold.

Healthy Rice Pudding
1 serving

Rice pudding is a healthy, well-known dish. It is used in many cuisines all around the world. It can be used as a dessert or as a main dish. Rice pudding's flaws are high calorie value and high amount of simple sugars. Both of those are not desirable in detoxification diets. That is why 'Healthy Rice Pudding' consists of high-quality rice, natural sweeteners, fruits, and spices. Made this way, it can be used as a part of many low fat, low-carb, or detox diets, as well as everyday meal.

1 cup of brown rice
4 ounces of low-fat milk
4 ounces of water
1 tablespoon of honey
1/2 teaspoon of maple syrup
1 teaspoon cinnamon powder
1 tablespoon coconut powder
1 tablespoon of blended Brazil nuts

Soak brown rice in 4 ounces of water. After 24 hours strain the water from the rice and again soak rice, this time in 4 ounces of milk. Leave it soaked for half a day. The longer the rice is soaked, the softer it will be. After that period add the rest of the ingredients into the mixture. Blend everything and put the pudding in the refrigerator and serve any time you want.

Eggplant with Cheese
1 serving

Eggplant is rich in nutrients, which eliminate free radicals. Combined with cheese, eggplant makes good source of quality carbohydrates and proteins.

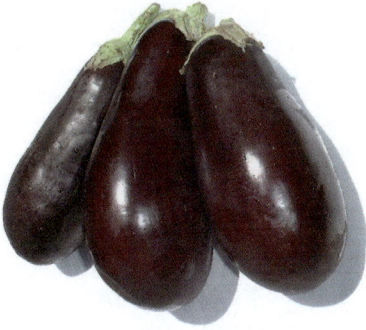

1 medium eggplant
6 ounces of low-fat cottage cheese
2 tablespoons of olive oil
Pinch of salt
1 tablespoon lemon juice
3-4 cloves of chopped garlic

Put whole eggplant (with skin) into boiling water and cook for 10 minutes. Move the eggplant into jar with cold water. After a while, peel the skin and crop the eggplant into several pieces. Sauté the pieces on olive oil for 5 minutes. Pour the lemon juice over sautéed eggplant and serve with mixture made from cheese and garlic.

Healthy Quince Cheese
1 serving

Traditional quince cheese is a highly caloric, fat, and sweet cake. During detox diet, people should avoid all of the mentioned properties of quince cheese. When you remove all of the unhealthy ingredients from traditional quince cheese recipe, you get 'Healthy Quince Cheese'. For this cake we use quince (which is used as a remedy for digestive system diseases), honey (natural sweetener, rich in various antioxidants), walnut (high amount of protein), and lemon (rich in vitamin C).

1 quince
1 lemon
3 tablespoons of honey
1 handful walnut

Put quince in boiling water and cook for 1 hour. After 1 hour drain water and add the honey and walnuts into the mixture. Cook for 10 to 15 minutes. During that time you need to stir the mass often. When it's done, let it cool for few hours and then serve.

Healthy Ice-cream
1 serving

During summer days, people often wish for something refreshing to help them cool. Many people seek solution in ice cream. It can invigorate the body for some period. However, there are very big problems regarding regular ice cream: high calorie value, simple sugars and fat. This recipe consists all of

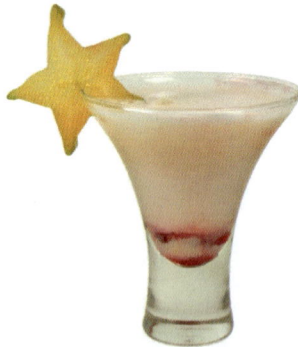

dietary ingredients, has low calorie value, and is rich in essential amino acids, vitamins, minerals and EFA.

5 ounces low-fat cottage cheese
2 ounces soymilk
1/2 medium banana
Handful of hazelnuts (chopped or whole)
Handful of blackcurrants
Handful of chokeberries
Handful of cranberries

Blend half a banana together with soymilk and cheese. Add the rest of the ingredients to the mixture and stir. Put it in freezer for several hours before serving.

Cream Pumpkin Soup
1 serving

Pumpkins are rich in essential nutrients, while poor in calories, and thus are often on diet menus. High amount of vitamins and minerals is the property of every ingredient in this soup. Pistachio nuts have the lowest calories of all nuts. This dish should certainly be consumed by those in need of vitamins A, C, B complex and potassium.

5 ounces of pumpkin flesh
1 onion
½ cup of fresh orange juice
½ cup of water
Pinch of ginger
1 tablespoon olive oil
Handful of chopped pistachio nuts

Sauté the onion in olive oil. Blend the pumpkin flesh until it becomes mushy. Add the pumpkin pulp to the pan and sauté for 5 minutes. Add equal amounts of water and orange juice to the mixture. Add ginger and pistachio nuts, and serve. Or blend everything together for a hot, soupy blend if on a liquid-detox fast.

Azuki and Pumpkin Soup
1 serving

This is a highly energizing soup that has majority of essential nutrients. Only one serving covers more than one third of recommended daily amounts of protein, vitamin A, potassium, and zinc. It is recommended for everyone on a detoxification diet. This soup can help heal some digestive problems.

1 cup azuki beans
1 cup blended pumpkin
3 cups water
1 tablespoon apple vinegar
1 teaspoon salt
1 chopped carrot
1 chopped onion
A pinch of pepper
½ teaspoon chili powder

Put all the ingredients into a pot and cook for two hours. Strain or puree.

Healthy Mary Cocktail
1 serving

This cocktail is based on the Bloody Mary cocktail, only without alcohol, sugar, and other unhealthy ingredients. Prepared in this way, the cocktail is healthy, fresh, and tasteful. It is rich in spices, which will accelerate body metabolism. It is best consumed in the morning to give strength and energy for the coming day.

Half a cup of fresh tomato juice
1 tablespoon lemon juice
A few black olives
Pinch of salt, pepper, saffron, horseradish powder, basil, chili pepper powder, ginger, and rosemary.

Puree all of the ingredients.

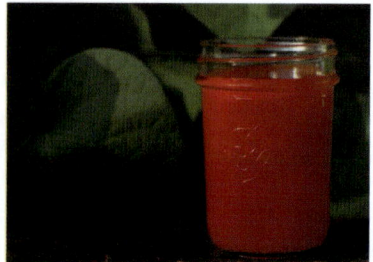

Soy Steak Recipe
1 serving

Soy is the richest plant in protein, it has high amount of minerals, fibers, and vitamins. That is why soy should be a regular meal in every detox diet. This dish is easy to digest thanks to yogurt bacteria. High amount of garlic makes this dish an immune system booster.

4 ounces of soy steak
4 ounces of yogurt
10 cloves of garlic
A pinch of salt and pepper
1 tablespoon olive oil
Handful parsley leaves

Add chopped garlic, salt, pepper, and parsley leaves to the yogurt. Chop soy stakes to get one square inch size pieces. Sauté the soy pieces in olive oil for 10 minutes. Pour the yogurt mixture over the soy and cook for another five minutes. When done, put in the refrigerator for 1 hour and serve cool – blended or 'chewing.'

Shitake Soup
1 serving

This recipe is made especially for those on detox diets for cancer, but everyone should include this dish in their menu as a precaution. Shitake mushrooms are proven tumor remedies; beetroot and chokeberries have plenty of different antioxidants, while citrus fruits are rich in vitamin C.

5 ounces shitake mushrooms
2 ounces beetroot

A pinch of salt
1 chopped onion
1 cup water
1 tablespoon fresh lemon juice
1 tablespoon fresh orange juice
1 tablespoon fresh grapefruit juice
Handful chokeberries

Boil beetroot for twenty minutes. Sauté the onion and after 5 minutes add shitake mushrooms. Grate the boiled beetroot into the pot. Shitake mushrooms should not be sautéd longer than two minutes. Sauté everything for two minutes, and then add a cup of water. Simmer for five minutes. When finished, add juices and chokeberries.

Wheat Germ and Nuts Dessert
1 serving

Wheat germ has 10% protein and mixed with various other types of nuts makes a tasty dessert high in protein, carbs, and essential fatty acids, all of which are necessary after extensive physical activity. This recipe can also be consumed by people who are on a diet that lacks protein. It will give body strength and energy, and won't produce any negative side effects. Every ingredient in the recipe has good detoxification qualities.

2 handfuls wheat germ
½ cup menthe tea
½ handful Brazil nuts
½ handful cashew nuts
½ handful almonds
½ handful dried banana chips
½ handful dried cranberries
2 tablespoons honey

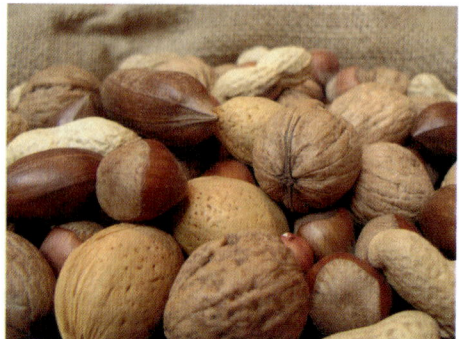

Warm menthe tea and add the honey in it. Stir it until honey dissolves. Pour over wheat germ, and add all of the nuts, banana chips, and cranberries. Blend or puree.

Wheat Grass Universal Drink
1 serving

Wheat grass contains every nutrient the body needs. It has a lot more vitamin C, vitamin B, carotene, and calcium than most other plants. It is very rich in proteins and fibers. Wheat grass drinks with lemon and honey are one prime natural remedy for all sorts of illnesses. Everyday use is recommended for everyone.

7 ounces of wheat seeds
1 tablespoon lemon juice
1 tablespoon honey
A few cups of water

Soak the wheat seeds in water for 24 hours in a covered jar. When germination appears, soak water and put seeds on a plate. Make sure that seeds get enough sunlight. Water it a bit every day. After a week grass should be few inches high. You should cut grass, wash it, and put it in blender, together with 8 ounces of water. Blend for several minutes. Add honey and lemon juice.

Daily Liver Cleanse
1 serving

If you are experiencing a general overall feeling of poor health, loss of sex drive, weakness and fatigue, anger, frustration, resentment, irritability and bitterness, you may be beginning to feel the problem

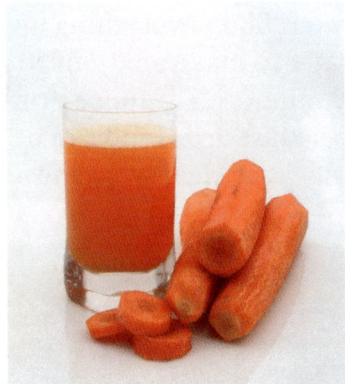

associated with elevated liver toxins. Here is a daily cleanse that will help return your liver to normal function.

1 cup warm water
1 tablespoon molasses
1 tablespoon extra virgin olive oil
2 tablespoons lemon juice
cayenne pepper to taste

Bring water to a boil and immediately remove from heat. Add molasses, lemon juice, olive oil and a pinch of cayenne (to taste). Drink this mixture first thing in the morning for 10 consecutive days.

Love Your Liver Herbal Detox Drink
1 serving

One way to restore balance to your liver and other internal organs is an aggressive, antioxidant drink. If you are just beginning your detox, you may want to try half of a serving to make sure you don't get overly dizzy from detox symptoms.

1 carrot,
1 beetroot
½ English cucumber
1 celery stalk

Wash all of the ingredients completely with distilled or purified water. Chop everything up and blend in a juicer. Add enough water to make an 8-ounce glass of juice. Drink the juice within 30 minutes. This juice drink is a good first-thing-in-the-morning breakfast drink and can be alternated for 10-days with another daily liver cleanse recipe.

Lean, Green Detox Machine
1 serving

This fatigue-prevention recipe is the Optimus Prime of detox drinks. Dark, green leafy vegetables are the highest in natural antioxidants. The apples add just a touch of sweetness.

1 medium red apple
1 stalk celery
1 broccoli floret
1 kale leaf
1 small handful of fresh parsley
1 collard leaf
1 carrot

Wash all of the ingredients completely with distilled or purified water. Chop everything up and blend in a juicer for an 8- to 12-ounce drink.

Fresh and Tangy
1 serving

3 carrots, topped
1 ounce wheatgrass juice (available at health foods store)
1 fresh lemon

Wash all of the ingredients completely with distilled or purified water. Remove the lemon peel. Dice all of the ingredients, blend and serve. OMG!

Broccoli and Watercress Soup
1 serving

Here is a great-tasting soup that allows the vegetables to stand out. It is very simple to make, and easy to modify with other vegetables to fit your individual taste.

½ tablespoon olive oil
½ clove garlic
¼ yellow onion
Half head broccoli
1-¼ cups water
Pinch each coarse salt
and freshly ground
black pepper to taste
½ cup fresh watercress
or arugula
1/3 lemon

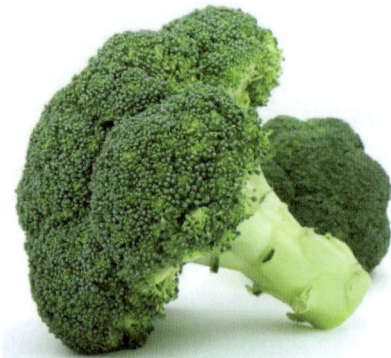

Thinly slice the garlic and lemon. Dice the onion and cut the broccoli into small florets. Heat the olive oil in a saucepan over medium heat. Add the garlic and onion and sauté for just about a minute. Add the broccoli and cook for about four minutes or until the broccoli is a bright green. Add the water, salt and pepper and bring everything to a boil. Lower the temperature and cover. Cook on low for eight minutes or until the broccoli is tender (6-7 minutes for al dente.) Pour the soup into a blender and puree with the watercress or the arugula until very smooth. Serve the soup topped off with a bit of the fresh lemon slices.

Root Juice Mix
1 serving

The liver is the main organ in body detoxification and that is why the liver suffers first. To help your liver maintain its function, we need to remove toxins from it. This recipe consists of different plant roots which have substances healthy for liver detox.

Besides the liver, this drink helps in detoxification of the kidneys and bowels.

1 ounce barberry root
1 ounce dandelion root
1 ounce Baikal skullcap (Scutellaria baicalensis) root
1 ounce bupleurum root
1 ounce blue flag (Iris missouriensis) root
1 ounce turmeric root
3 ounces boiling water
3 ounces fresh orange juice
3 ounces whey

Pour boiling water over the blended roots. Let it rest for 24 hours. Strain the juice from it and mix the juice with orange juice and whey.

Triple Action Drink
1 serving

Toxins accumulate mostly in your liver, kidneys, and bowels. This drink contains ingredients that affect all three organs. Parsley is a powerful diuretic and helps in kidney detoxification; rucola is rich in vitamin C and has nutrients that help liver detox; apple will give the drink sweetness and good taste, and provide fibers necessary for bowel cleansing.

2 teaspoons minced parsley
2 teaspoons minced rucola (Eruca sativa) leaves
1 apple
8 ounces mint tea

Blend apple and mix with other ingredients. Let it sit for half an hour before consuming.

Morning Drink
1 serving

The 'Morning Drink' will boost bodily functions that were slowed during sleep. It will supply the body with necessary carbohydrates, protein, minerals, and vitamins. Black tea contains caffeine which is a stimulant, so this drink can be used as a substitute for coffee.

1 handful flax seeds
1 handful wheat germ
1 tablespoon fresh orange juice
2 black tea bags
1 tablespoon cocoa powder
1 tablespoon honey (optional)
4 ounces soy milk
5 ounces of boiling water

Blend flax seeds and wheat germ to make powder. Make the tea - pour boiling water over tea bags and cocoa. After 5 minutes remove the teabags and add flax seed and germ powder. Stir the mixture and add soy milk. Depending on your preference, this drink can be used chilled or hot.

Milk Thistle Tea
1 serving

This is one of the most powerful drinks for whole-body detoxification. It is especially effective for liver detox. The tea will help the body to release toxins accumulated in liver, kidneys, bowels, and blood. It is recommended for everyone who has a toxic liver or has used a lot of alcohol and unhealthy food.

1 tablespoon milk thistle seeds
1 tablespoon parsley leaves

4 ounces boiling water
1 tablespoon lemon
1 ounce fresh orange juice
3 ounces chamomile tea
3 ounces mint tea

Pour boiling water over the milk thistle seeds. Leave for 5 minutes before straining it. Mix the milk thistle tea with orange juice chamomile and mint tea. Add parsley leaves. It can be served either hot or cooled.

Digestion Mix
1 serving

Detox drink designed primary for bowel detoxification, but also helps detoxification of other organs. It can be used as a remedy for bad digestion, lack of stomach acid, abdominal bloating, and constipation. Plums are rich in fibers that improve digestion, while spices accelerate metabolism. Mild properties of yogurt will soothe every part of the digestive system.

3-5 plums
7 ounces yogurt
1/3 teaspoon rosemary
1/3 teaspoon ginger
1/3 teaspoon cinnamon
1/3 teaspoon cloves
1/3 teaspoon cayenne pepper powder
1/3 teaspoon oregano
1 tablespoon pumpkin seeds
1 tablespoon honey

Put everything in blender and blend until it gets mushy. Put the mix in your freezer to cool a bit before serving.

Night Drink
1 serving

Lack of sleep is in many cases the main cause of illness. This detoxification recipe includes ingredients that improve a night's sleep. Healthy, natural sleep is of great importance during your detox diet. This drink should be used by everyone, but especially by those who are in need of rest. Besides having anti-stress properties 'Night Drink' is rich in antioxidants, vitamins, and minerals that will help the immune system.

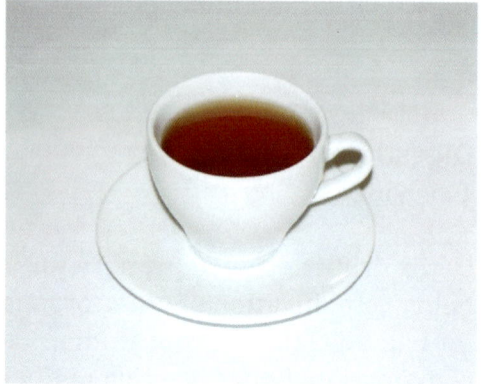

7 ounces low-fat milk
½ medium banana
1 ounce of boiling water
1 tablespoon St John's wort
½ teaspoon anise
1 teaspoon chopped walnuts
2 teaspoons sour cherry juice
1 tablespoon sesame

Make banana shake of milk and half a banana. Pour boiling water over St John's wort and anise. Add it to the banana shake. Finally, blend or grind up and add the walnuts, sesame, and cherry juice to the mix. Drink before going to bed.

Anti-Stress Mix
1 serving

During a diet people suffer both physical and mental stress. The main attribute of this drink is its detoxification property, but this drink also has nutrients that affect mood and fight stress. Drink this beverage whenever you feel depressed, tired, or after extensive physical activity. A combination of asparagus and poppy seeds give it an extraordinary taste. Use honey to sweeten this peculiar drink.

1 tablespoon poppy seed powder
1/2 tablespoon cocoa powder
1 handful of chopped asparagus shoots
1 blended carrot
1 handful of chopped almonds
4 ounces of fresh orange juice
4 ounces chamomile tea
2 tablespoons honey

Dry roast or bake the poppy seeds for ten minutes. Pour chamomile tea over it and add cocoa powder. Cook for ten more minutes. When done, put in the freezer to cool for twenty minutes. After that period, add the rest of the ingredients to the mixture.

Leaf Tea
1 serving

The recipe consists of various sorts of plant leaves. All of the ingredients have in common powerful detoxification properties. Leaves will give the tea peculiar taste, while honey will provide sweetness. Mixed all together, it makes powerful weapon for elimination of toxins from the body.

1 tablespoon artichoke leaves
1 tablespoon raspberry leaves
1 tablespoon bladderwrack leaves
1 tablespoon beet leaves
1 tablespoon parsley leaves
2 tablespoon honey
8 ounces boiling water

Pour the boiling water over the mixed leaves. Strain after 5 minutes, than add honey. If you prefer ice-tea, put the tea in freezer for 20 minutes.

Digestion Help
1 serving

During your detox diet some people can have digestive problems, especially in the beginning, while still adapting to the new nutrition. This drink will help remedy bloating, gastritis, and ease the digestive tract. It is effective in treating every gastric problem and has liver detox properties. Parsley is particularly good for kidney detox, because of its diuretic attributes.

1 tablespoon chamomile
1 tablespoon anise
1 tablespoon star gentian
1 tablespoon mint
1 tablespoon centaury plant flower
8 ounces of boiling water
1 tablespoon lemon juice
1 tablespoon honey
1 tablespoon parsley

Pour the boiling water over chamomile, anise, star gentian, mint, and centaury plant flower. After 5 minutes, strain. Add lemon juice, honey, and parsley to the tea.

Strong Drink
1 serving

Although this drink has relatively low calorie value it will give the body strength. It is rich in nutrients that act as a stimulus, so it should be consumed every time you're feeling weak or depressed. All of the ingredients are rich in vitamins and minerals. This drink is good for every detox diet because of its antioxidant substances.

½ teaspoon guarana extract
1 tablespoon lemon juice
1 tablespoon royal jelly
1 tablespoon honey
1 handful strawberries
5 ounces pineapple
5 ounces orange juice

Blend all the ingredients together. It makes even more refreshing drink when served cold or over ice.

Self-Talk – Daily Spiritual, Mental and Emotional Affirmations to Help You in Your Journey

There is no doubt about it. Making such a life change is difficult. Even with the encouragement of friends and family, when the lights go out and the noises dissipate, you're the only one there and you're going through the process alone. This section of the book is here to help you get through times of doubt, worry, discouragement and depression. You can be your own worst enemy, or your own best friend. Come on! Let's all be friends!

Read each of the daily anecdotes and affirmations. They're there to encourage and uplift you. I know you'll feel better.

Also, here is a short list of questions for you to keep a journal every day. This will also help you see where you've been, where you are and help you understand where you're going. What are your experiences? How do you feel? Are you meeting your goal?

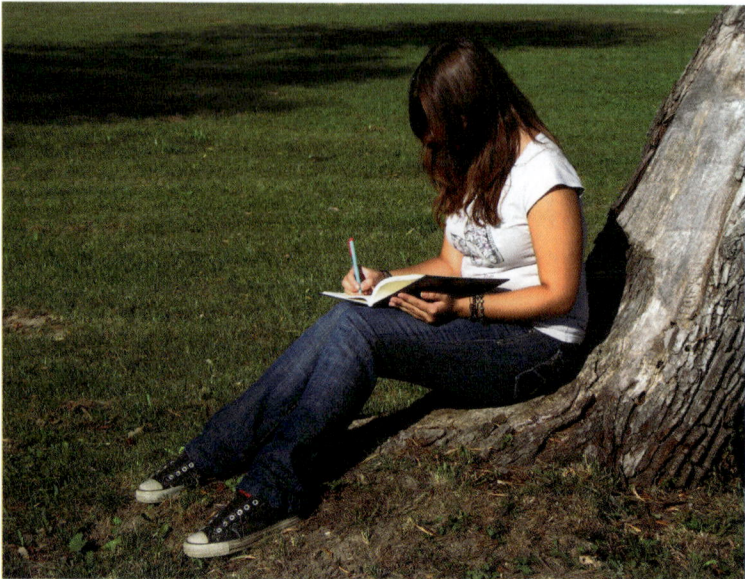

Keep track of thoughts, ideas and experiences that will help you the next go-around.

> How do I feel today?
> How much do I weigh?
> How much weight have I lost?
> What changes have I noticed in my physical well-being?
> How has my mental self changed?
> What spiritual changes am I experiencing?
> What are my goals for today?

Let's get started!

Day 1)

Changing our poor habits and maintaining a positive and healthy lifestyle is a powerful decision to make. However, this life-changing decision can sometimes come along with distractions, negative thoughts, and wanting to give up. It is easy and common to feel overwhelmed when making a huge lifestyle change. Don't let negative feelings overpower you when you are struggling or feel like you're having a bad day. Get up and go, push the negativity aside, and start to focus on the good things in life, such as losing weight, staying healthy, and living longer.

Use the following daily affirmation to help you achieve your weight goals and maintain a positive attitude:

I am strong and I have made a positive choice to change my lifestyle in a healthier way. I know I will face obstacles, I know I will have fears, and I know this will be a difficult road to travel, but I will not let anything get in my way of achieving my goals. I am healthy, I am positive, and I deserve the best.

Day 2)

You want to see yourself as a thinner, healthier, and more energetic person. Maybe you have young children that enjoy outdoor activities, such as riding bicycles, going to the park, or swimming. You want to enjoy these activities with them, share the fun times, and create everlasting memories. Eating healthier and maintaining a healthier weight will give you more energy and allow you to participate with ease in your children's daily activities. Participating in these activities with your children is also a wonderful way to encourage healthy behavior, by staying active.

To help you achieve your weight loss goals, use this daily affirmation to remind you of the importance of your goals and the rewards you will receive by achieving them:

I have children who need me in their lives. I do not want to miss anything that they achieve in life. I know if I achieve my weight loss goals, I will be healthier, live longer, and I can participate in activities that involve my children and exercise. I will challenge myself by participating in their outdoor activities daily. I will encourage myself and my children to enjoy being and staying active, as a family.

Day 3)

You are aiming to lose weight, eat healthier, and maintain an active lifestyle. You know what you have to do to achieve these goals, but you also know the road may get "bumpy". We all make mistakes, we all get frustrated, and sometimes we don't always perform at 100%. One of the most important things to keep you on track is to give yourself some credit! You've made a life changing decision to live a healthier lifestyle and set weight loss goals! This is one of the hardest decisions in life you have ever made. Focus on the positive things you have done with your goals. Maybe you have consistently had a healthy breakfast each morning or you have maintained 30 minutes of exercise daily, these are all great things! If you make one mistake, do not beat yourself up; instead, think about the positive and how you can move on.

To help you stay positive and remind yourself that it is important to give yourself credit and focus on the benefits of your goals, use the following affirmation daily:

I have made a goal to lose weight and stay active. I might make a mistake, but I am human. I will not let a mistake or negative thought stop me from my goals. If I miss an exercise date or give into a temptation, I will not beat myself up for it. I will remind myself that I am strong; I can overcome temptations and laziness. I will move forward, focusing on the future of healthy living and not focusing on my past mistakes. In every failure, there is an opportunity. I am a winner and I will succeed.

Day 4)

In addition to maintaining an exercise routine and eating healthy, there are plenty of things you can do to throughout the day to stay active. Some people like to say, "Start small" when it comes you to goals. You have set your goals to lose weight to improve your overall health. Don't feel like you should limit yourself to certain things. Remember that this is an overall lifestyle and body change! Instead of "starting small", add some "small" things to your daily routine that will increase your energy and help you get closer to your weight loss goals.

Use this affirmation daily to remind yourself of the different things you can do each day to help yourself achieve a healthy and ideal weight:

I know that I will exercise daily and maintain a healthy meal plan. I know that this will lead me to my ideal weight. I can challenge myself every day by doing small things to keep me active. I will make my bed every morning. I will park my car at least 10 car spots away from any building rather than looking for the closest spot. I will use the stairs and not the elevator. I will carry the grocery bags from the store rather than use a cart. I will stretch during my favorite TV show. I can do any of these things daily and I know it will help me get closer to my goal.

Day 5)

You have made a goal to lose weight to improve your overall health. Eating well-balanced and nutritious meals are very important to achieving your goal. It is also important to include daily exercise in to your routine, to help you reach your goal. One very important element in losing weight is the addition of water to your diet. You know that adding water throughout your day will keep you hydrated, keep you feeling fuller longer, and increase your immune system. Staying healthy while losing weight is very important, getting sick can easily push you off track from reaching your goals. Water is crucial in keeping you on track and losing weight while staying healthy.

To reach your weight loss goals in a safe and healthy manner, use this daily affirmation:

I will shape my own future and I will take control of where my life is going. I will stay healthy while reaching my goals. I know that drinking water daily is very important to remaining healthy and also in losing weight. I will replace my soda with water. I will drink at least 8 ounces of water per day. I will carry a water bottle with me at all times. I am dedicated, I am confident, and I enjoy water because it is good for me and will help me reach my goals.

Day 6)

We know that restaurants and fast food chains serve us portions that are much, much more than we actually need. You want to lose weight and one way to do so is by eating healthy. Healthy food is important and so are healthy portion sizes. You know that the hungrier you are, the more you will eat. You can fight this urge to overeat by replacing regular dining room size plates (usually 10-14") with salad plates (usually 7-9"). By using smaller plates for your meals, you will be able to have a full plate and a normal, healthy size portion, thus, one more step to getting closer to your ideal weight!

Use the following daily affirmation to remind you of healthy portion sizes for your weight loss goal:

I enjoy a well-balanced meal. I enjoy a full plate and I deserve a full plate because I have been working hard towards my weight loss goals. I will use smaller, salad sized plates for my meals, so that I can have a full plate and know that I am not overeating. Not only will I be rewarding myself with a healthy and nutritious meal, I will not feel like I am starving myself, because I will have a full plate. This is the right size portion I should be eating and it will make me thin, healthy, and happy.

Day 7)

Making a plan and sticking to it can be difficult and lonely. You have made a goal to lose weight to live a longer, happier, and healthier life. While we will all agree that it is easy to make the goal, it can be hard to stick to it when you are doing it by yourself. Motivation is a key factor in achieving success. Find a friend, family member, or co-worker who is also interested in improving their lifestyle. Even if they do not have the exact same goals as you do, you can find ways to incorporate your individual healthy lifestyle goals in a manner that can motivate both of you and keep you on track.

If you have a family member who is interested in exercising, set a time for every day, at the exact same time, to meet up and exercise. Knowing that someone else is counting on you to be there can be a wonderful motivator. If you have a co-worker who is looking to improve their diet, plan your meals together and have lunch daily. Simple things like this will help you achieve your goals and at the same time, you will be helping another person achieve their goals as well.

Use the following affirmation to remind yourself that we all need motivation and sometimes friends and family members can be the best answer:

I am motivated. I am a motivator. I will make sure I have someone in my life, daily, who is motivating me and I am motivating them. I will not let them down and I will not let myself down. I will meet them at the gym every morning, I will have a healthy lunch with them every day, or I will take an evening walk with them every night. Every time I motivate someone else, they in turn motivate me to reach my goal. I can do it. We can do it.

Day 8)

Bad habits need not stick around. We know you do not put yourself in situations where you might slip back into unhealthy habits or temptations. You don't see a recovering alcoholic working as a bartender. You don't see an ex-smoker hanging out with the smokers outside at lunch break. This goes the same for you and your weight loss goals. You are more likely to be tempted to eat fatty foods if you go to fast food restaurants. It's not easy to go to a fast food restaurant, smell the French fries and the hamburgers on the grill, and then easily order a salad. Anybody would be tempted in that situation! So avoid fast food restaurants, avoid the inner aisles of the grocery market (where most of the bad food is located), and avoid people who might bring you down or help you fall into your old ways. This is your life, you control it and you know that by surrounding yourself with positives will help you reach your health goals much faster.

Repeat this daily affirmation when you find yourself being tempted by old or bad habits:

I have chosen a healthy lifestyle and made weight loss goals so that I can live longer, feel more energetic, and look better. I will not go to fast food restaurants. I will not indulge in happy hour. I will plan my meals every day. If I have to eat at a restaurant, I will choose a restaurant with healthy choices. I will not miss my old habits; they are unhealthy and they stop me from reaching my health goals. I will lose weight, I will be healthy, and I am on track.

Day 9)

You know that healthy food is essential to losing weight. There is a reason why Doctors stress that children eat their fruits and vegetables starting at a young age. Fruits and vegetables contain so many vital nutrients and minerals to keeping us healthy, fighting illness, preventing cancer, and also maintaining a healthy waistline. Use these healthy foods to help bulk up your food. Increasing the amount of vegetables in your stir-fry or your pasta salad, can actually allow you to eat twice the amount of food for half the calories of the normal, restaurant-style stir-fry or pasta salad. Including extra vegetables and fruits into your meals can also help you feel fuller longer. You will not have mid-morning, mid-afternoon, or even late night junk food cravings. By just adding more fruits and vegetables to your daily menu, you will move faster towards your goal of losing weight and maintaining a healthy waistline.

Use this affirmation daily to remind you that fruits and vegetables are essential to reaching your weight loss goals:

I know that healthy foods will help me lose weight. I will add vegetables and fruits to every meal I make every day. I will find enjoyment in learning new healthy recipes and snacks that I can incorporate vegetables and fruits in. I will even try vegetables and fruits that I have never tried before. I will feel satisfied, I will feel full, and I will know that what I am consuming is healthy for my body and will help me towards reaching my ideal weight.

Day 10)

You know that sugar is bad for you. You know that eating sugary foods, white breads, potatoes, and white pasta will decrease your odds of losing weight. There are so many different options available nowadays in public grocery stores that feature healthier versions of these "white" foods. Whole grain breads, brown rice, and whole wheat pasta are wonderful substitutions for those "white" and starchy foods that you crave. Introduce these new foods to your family in a fun way. Try new recipes. As with everything, some things take getting used to. You will know that this major change in the types of starches or carbohydrates that you and your family consume will not only help you towards your goal of weight loss, but these foods will benefit your entire family's health and well-being as well.

Read this daily affirmation to yourself when shopping or preparing your meals to remind you of the good foods to consume when losing weight:

I know there are healthier options to foods like pasta, bread, and rice. I will look forward to trying new foods. I will only purchase whole grain bread, whole wheat pasta, and brown rice for my kitchen pantry. I will welcome and embrace these new foods because they are helping me reach my goal of weight loss and a healthy lifestyle. These whole grain foods are beneficial to my overall health as well as the health of my family.

Day 11)

Eating can be an emotional outlet for some people. Remind yourself that emotional eating can lead to overeating. Remember that you have made a goal to better yourself, lose weight, and live a healthier lifestyle. Enjoy your meals because they are healthy, taste delicious, and most importantly, you made them. Take time to enjoy, eat slowly, and calmly. Chew each bite of food at least 10-20 times. Let your brain be aware of what you are putting into your body so that you have time to feel full. Cleanse your pallet frequently with water, have conversation with your family or dinner guests, and appreciate this moment of healthy eating.

Repeat this daily affirmation before or during meals to yourself so you can take full advantage of wholesome eating:

I will enjoy my food but eat slowly and calmly. I will let my brain catch up with me while I eat by putting my spoon or fork down between bites, having conversations with my family, and frequently cleansing my pallet with sips of water. This will help me enjoy my food, eat the right amount of food, and feel satisfied. It is ok for me to enjoy eating when I appreciate each bite. I am on the right track; I am reaching my goal to weight loss success.

Day 12)

You know that you need to stay away from old and bad habits in order to achieve your goal of losing weight. You most likely have friends and family members who you once shared these bad habits with when going out for social events or entertaining. You can still have your night out; just make sure it is an outing that is filled with healthy activity. Instead of going to the local bar for happy hour, ask your girlfriends to join you for an evening Zumba class or your buddies to a game of racquet ball at the local YMCA. Not only will you get an amazing workout, you and your friends will have an amazing time!

Read this affirmation to remind you that there are still plenty of options to have fun with your friends when achieving your weight loss goal:

I can still have fun. My weight loss goals do not hinder my social life. I am an energetic individual. I will opt for evening or weekend activities that allow me to be physically active and have fun at the same time. This will benefit me physically, mentally, and emotionally. I will be social in a positive way. I will enjoy walking through the park, taking a dancing class, or going on a bike ride. These activities release endorphins throughout my body, making me feel good and they offer great physical rewards. This is my social enjoyment and I love it.

Day 13)

You deserve the best. So does your family. You know that it is important to your family for you to be healthy and to live a long life. Remember that both you and your family deserve the best. Understand that this situation is not forever. Do not limit yourself because you feel that you do not deserve something due to your current situation. If you have lost 10 pounds and your goal is to lose 50lbs, get excited about this and all the possibilities that lay ahead. Reward yourself! Donate the clothes that are in your closet and do not fit you. Buy yourself a new pair of pants or a new shirt. Congratulate yourself for every milestone that you reach. This will keep you on track, get you excited, and show your family that you are making a conscious effort and the results are showing.

Use this affirmation to remind yourself that you deserve to be healthy and rewarded:

I am winning. I am making progress. I am working towards my goals and it is showing. I am thinner, I am healthier, and I am happier. I deserve rewards, I deserve to be successful, and I deserve to be thin and healthy.

Day 14)

Late night cravings can be your worst enemy when trying to lose weight. Don't let this bad habit affect your goal of weight loss. Make a rule to both yourself and your family that the kitchen closes after 7pm. Stick to lunch and dinner recipes that will feed you and your entire family with the appropriate portions. If you have a recipe for lasagna that makes 12 servings but you have a family of 6, cut the recipe in half. This will help avoid leftovers, which can be the culprit of late night eating. If there are no leftovers in the refrigerator, then there is a less likely possibility that you will be tempted to raid the fridge late at night. Eating past dinner time will increase the amount of calories you intake for the day and delay you from reaching your weight loss goal. If you absolutely need something to snack on and it is past dinner time, allow yourself a low calorie, healthy, and vitamin-rich food such as a banana, which will actually help prepare you for morning exercise!

I know that my body needs at least 3 healthy meals and 2 healthy snacks per day in order for me to reach my weight loss and fitness goals. I will not eat past dinner time. By doing this, I will only set myself back in reaching my goals. I will make sure not to skip meals or snacks. By eating at my designated time in the morning, afternoon, and evening, I will be satisfied throughout the day and not be tempted to snack late at night. I am disciplined and I will achieve my goals to weight loss.

Day 15)

You know that sometimes nutritious and healthy foods may taste bland at first, especially if you are used to eating a greasy and salty diet. Using the appropriate amounts of spices, herbs, and sauces in your daily meals can really add some life to your new and healthy cuisine. Some spices can even reduce your appetite, such as hot peppers. Add some hot peppers or Cayenne pepper to the sauce you use on your pasta, your stir fry, and even your chili. Get creative with your cooking but remember that some condiments and dressings may look healthy, but dousing your salad with more than 1-2 tablespoons can make the calories add up quickly. Remember that you can enjoy healthy food with just a hint of spices, dressings, or healthy fats.

Review this affirmation daily when you cook at home or eat out at restaurants to help ensure you meet your weight loss goals:

I am proud to be cooking and consuming healthy meals. They are helping me reach my weight loss goals. I am losing weight and getting thinner. I will remember to use salad dressings, condiments, and healthy fats sparingly. I enjoy the healthy taste of eating natural fruits and vegetables. They come from the earth and they are good for me. I can be creative and cook exotic and delicious meals without using high calorie sweeteners and condiments. I am an amazing cook and I am amazing at my goals.

Day 16)

Things happen in life that either get in the way of your "ideal" plan or disrupt your daily schedule. Instead of making excuses for not following your plan to lose weight and get healthy, focus on finding the solution to the problem. You might not be able to make your daily gym visit if your child has to stay home from school because he/she is sick. Don't let this stop you from your goals. So you can't make it to the gym today but you can still find ways to stay active. Vacuum the entire house, scrub your floors, do an at-home circuit session in your family room, or even wash your car (if the weather permits of course). Remember that things will disrupt your life often, but do not let them stop you from accomplishing your goals. There is always an alternative to a plan that has been interrupted.

Read this daily affirmation when you feel like your plan for the day has been altered:

I have a goal to lose weight and get healthy. I will not let the small things in life deter me from reaching this goal. If something happens that I may not have expected, I must remember that there is always a solution to a problem. I will not make excuses. I will not stray from my goal. I will improvise and compromise to achieve my ultimate goal of losing weight, getting thin, and living life.

Day 17)

You know now the difference between what is healthy and what is un-healthy when it comes to the foods that we put into our body. However, certain nutrients and minerals that can be found in foods are very important for us to be aware of because they are essential for weight loss, a healthy digestive system, and an overall healthy body. One of the most important nutrients we can consume on a daily basis is fiber. Both soluble and insoluble fibers are beneficial to our bodies because they help correct our digestive system, reduce cholesterol levels, prevent certain forms of cancer, and fiber makes us feel full! You should consume at least 25 grams of fiber each day to reap all the benefits it has to offer.

Review this daily affirmation to help you reach your weight loss goal in a healthy and natural way:

Fiber is an essential nutrient that my body needs in order to lose weight and stay healthy. I will consume at least 5 servings of fruit and vegetables, as well as some servings of whole grain products, every day. Including fiber into my daily diet will not only help me reach my weight loss goals, it will also be beneficial to protecting my health and overall body well-being.

Day 18)

Your life may seem to get busier every day. In order to get all your tasks accomplished in the day, it may be easy to tell yourself that "it's ok to skip this meal, I'll just eat later." Eating three meals day and at least two healthy snacks is essential to you reaching your goal of weight loss. The most important meal of the day, and you have probably heard this from your doctor, is breakfast. Never skip breakfast. This is the meal that fuels your body and prepares it for the day. In order to achieve your goal of reaching your ideal weight, make sure you make breakfast a meal that is filled with protein and complex carbs to help you feel energized and ready to take on the day!

This affirmation can be read daily to remind you that breakfast is one of the most important elements to you reaching your weight loss goals:

Breakfast is the most important meal of the day. It fuels me and gives me energy to tackle everything that life throws at me during the day. I will never skip breakfast. I will make sure my breakfast is healthy and an appropriate portion. Breakfast will help me get thin. Breakfast will start my day off on the right foot. Breakfast is good.

Day 19)

You know that preparing three healthy meals a day is essential to your goal of weight loss. It is also very important to allow yourself 2-3 snacks a day to fight hunger cravings that may lead to a fast food binge. Keep healthy snacks with you at all times. These snacks can be a small bag or container of salad, apples, celery and peanut butter, grapes, etc. It may also be a wise idea for you to purchase your healthy snacks and then divide them into "snack-size" portions at home, keep them in small bags, and store in your refrigerator or pantry. This way they are easy, on-the-go snacks, handy, and very healthy. Most importantly, you will not be tempted to hit the vending machine at work or the drive-thru while running errands.

Read this daily affirmation to remind you that snacks are incredibly important to your goal of weight loss:

In order for me to reach my weight loss goals, I must have at least 2-3 healthy snacks a day. I will keep healthy snacks on me or within close proximity at all times. I will not be tempted by fast food, vending machines, or convenience store junk food. Healthy snacks taste better, they are better for me, and they will help me become thinner.

Day 20)

You know you have a sweet tooth but also know that indulging in desserts can set you back on your goal to lose weight. It is ok to have a dessert after dinner every now and then, but you can actually satisfy your sweet tooth in healthier and less caloric ways. Instead of having a slice of red velvet cake, have a small piece of dark chocolate and fruit. You can also relieve some of those sweet cravings by sipping on some sparkling water with lemon, raspberries, or lime. Sipping on water or fruit flavored sparkling water during times of sugar cravings, can actually decrease the craving within 5-10 minutes. Give it a try and you will save on those hefty calories of desserts like cake and ice cream.

Think twice about dessert and read this affirmation daily:

I enjoy sweet foods, but I do not need them every day. I can treat myself to dessert when it is appropriate. I can eat fruit every day. I can fight my sugar cravings with sparkling water and fruit. I am strong and superior to cravings. I am thinner and I am successful. I am reaching my goals.

Day 21)

Soda is one of the worst things you can consume. It is even worse when you are consuming it and allow your children to consume it. Soda contains enormous amounts of sugar. It is one of the primary causes of obesity, diabetes, and even tooth-decay. You do not want this for your family or for yourself. Worst of all, is that many people think diet soda is a good replacement for regular soda. It is in fact worse than regular soda. Replace soda with homemade lemonade and flavored water. Your family will love it and so will your waistline.

Review this affirmation daily when thinking about the healthy choices you can make in your household:

Both soda and diet soda are detrimental to my family's health as well as my own. I cannot reach my weight loss goals with soda in my diet. I will not drink soda or diet soda. I will enjoy water, flavored water, and even homemade lemonade every day. I will hydrate myself with these natural and delicious drinks. My family will be healthier. I will be healthier. I am now closer to my weight loss goal.

Day 22)

Sometimes, even after following your 3 meal and 2 snacks a day diet plan, you may still feel abnormally hungry before a meal. This may be due to stress or even a trigger such as the smells from a restaurant, popcorn cooking in the office break room, or seeing an advertisement on TV. An easy way to fight off these hunger pains is to drink an 8 ounce glass of water approximately 15-20 minutes before your meal. This will help you stay on track; eat only the meal portion you have prepared, and you will feel more satisfied in the end. Remember that water is one of the most important and essential elements in weight loss and overall health. Incorporate it as much as you can in your daily routine.

To fight hunger and unhealthy food cravings, review this daily affirmation:

I will not succumb to hunger cravings. I am strong and powerful. I do not want unhealthy, fatty, or greasy foods. My goal is to get better, thinner, and healthier. I will fight my hunger cravings with water. Water is crucial for me to lose weight. I will fail with unhealthy food. I will succeed with water.

Day 23)

Eating healthy and maintaining a regular exercise routine is essential to you in losing weight. You know that without those two requirements, you will not reach your goal. However, even by eating healthy and going to the gym daily, you may be limiting yourself. If you work a desk job all day long, get some extra activity throughout the day rather than lounging on your bum. Take a few 10-minute breaks throughout the day and climb a few stairs, walk around the office, or even try some seated leg and arm exercises. By doing this throughout the day, you will not only notice more pounds being shed, but it can actually help you feel more energized and stimulated at work.

Remember that you can always sneak in extra physical activity by reading this daily affirmation:

I am not restricted to one workout routine a day. I will make a conscious effort to get up throughout the day and take 10 minutes to do some sort of physical activity. I will not be a couch potato. I will not sit at my desk all day. Sitting all day is actually detrimental to my health as well as my weight loss goals. I will be active as often as possible and I will be thin.

Day 24)

You won't reach your weight loss goals with a negative attitude. You may be held back from reaching your goals if you have negative friends. The point is, make positive thinking a habit and surround yourself with positive people. By being positive, you will directly and indirectly encourage yourself and the people around you. Make positive thinking an everyday occurrence whether you're in a good or bad mood. You will reach your weight loss goals in an easier and smoother fashion this way.

Review this daily affirmation to remind yourself of the importance of positive thinking:

The success of my weight loss goal is based upon my attitude. I will lose weight and maintain a healthy lifestyle only with a positive attitude. I will only surround myself with people who are positive. I will maintain a goal-oriented environment at all times. Regardless of if I am in a good or bad mood, I will strive to continue a positive attitude. My positive attitude is the key to success for losing weight.

Day 25)

It is ok to rest. You have been working so hard with maintaining a healthy diet and workout routine that you have to remind yourself that your body still needs rest. Depending on the intensity of your workout and muscle soreness, make sure that you rotate the muscles you exercise every 1-3 days. You need to give muscles time to rest; otherwise, you may end up with an injury which could cause you to have to stop exercising all together until you are healed.

Review this daily affirmation in regards to your exercise routine and rest:

I am exercising regularly. I am getting stronger. I must remind myself that I should not push myself to the limits for fast results, this could lead to injury. I will get the appropriate rest needed after an intense work out. I will rotate my exercise routine. I am losing weight and I am gaining control over my body.

Day 26)

Distractions can be a major pitfall when it comes to completing anything in life. You know that your weight loss plan needs your full attention and you cannot be distracted by any means. When you eat, you should not be distracted. This could lead to over-eating and reaching for the wrong foods. Make it a rule in your household that the TV goes off during dinner time and that food is not allowed in the TV room. In addition to this, if you plan on going to see a movie with your friends or family, make sure you eat dinner BEFORE heading out or bring a healthy snack like carrots or grapes with you. Entertainment distractions can be the worst when it comes to losing weight, so stand firm and lose the tube when it comes to meal time.

Read this daily affirmation regarding distractions and your weight loss goal:

Distractions will deter me from reaching my goals. I will not eat with the television on. I will not allow food to be consumed in the family room or living room. Meal time is for consuming healthy food and enjoying time with friends and family. I will fight distractions and overcome them. I am winning my battle with weight and I am thin. I will not lose to my distractions.

Day 27)

Write it down. You will be understand, appreciate, and be more mindful of your weight loss plan and healthy eating if you keep a journal. Keep track of your daily workouts, your activities, your meals and calories. Noticing these things over time will give you a better idea of what works for you and what doesn't. It is also a great way to motivate you by writing down your thoughts and goals. Seeing things in ink on paper is sometimes easier to believe and act upon than just thinking about them in your head. After a few days you will be able to see all the healthy choices you have made and the things you need to work on for your weight loss to be truly successful.

Read this daily affirmation to understand the importance of keeping a journal:

I understand that in order to see my progress, I need to track it as well. I will keep a daily journal to track the food I eat, the activities I do, my daily mood, as well as my weight loss progress. I will monitor my overall growth to reward myself with the healthy choices I make as well as to see how I can improve my progress. I am getting healthier, losing weight, and feeling great.

Day 28)

A healthy lifestyle and weight loss plan is not just 5 days a week. This is a lifestyle change and only you can make it happen. It is ok to entertain or relax on the weekends however you can still have fun by enjoying yourself in a healthy way. Whenever you have free time, remember that how you spend it will affect your weight loss goals. If you can't make it to the gym, do any kind of activity that involves moving around like walking, raking the yard, or swimming. Choose activities that allow you to maintain your healthy diet plan as well. If you attend a BBQ, bring some healthy side dishes for the host of the party. This way you have options if the food that the host is cooking is not part of your meal plan. Don't stop your progress of achieving weight loss because of two "relaxation" days every week. Enjoy the weekends but spend them wisely.

Read the following affirmation daily to understand how you can use weekends in a beneficial way for your weight loss plan:

I will enjoy and reward myself during the weekend. I will choose to do so in a healthy and physically active manner. I will continue to eat nutritiously and maintain a form of exercise during my 2 day weekend every week. By approaching weekends in this fashion, I am getting closer to my ideal weight and enjoying a healthier lifestyle.

Day 29)

Losing weight and changing your lifestyle can be really stressful. This does not help as stress has been known to actually cause weight gain. If you feel stressed during your weight loss plan, remember that the stress will not go away by using food as comfort or sleep as a way to avoid the stress. Look at things with fresh eyes and try not to stress. Remember that things are not as bad as they seem and that there is always a solution or resolution in the end. It's not the end of the world. Surround yourself with positive people and environments and you will feel less stressed and see the pressure you feel on your shoulders will start to diminish. If you find yourself in a stressful situation try relaxing by doing something for yourself, go to the park or beach, watch a funny movie or television show, or take a bike ride and relax your mind as you view the local scenery. You can overcome stress and continue on with your weight loss plan easily with the right mindset.

The following daily affirmation will remind you of how to deal with stress during your weight loss plan:

I will not let stress take over my life or stop me from reaching my weight loss goals. I am in control of my body and my mind. If I feel stressed, I will take time to myself, relax, and do an activity that is peaceful. Surrounding myself with positive people and a positive environment will help me avoid stress and help me move forward with my weight loss goals. I am stronger than stress and it will not run my life.

Day 30)

Understanding the health benefits of weight loss is probably the most important thing to know when you start or follow a weight loss plan. Overweight women have a high risk of developing diabetes and overweight men have a risk of developing fatal heart problems. The risks of cancer, heart attacks, and other illnesses increase as we get older. If you have a family that cares about you or if you have goals and aspirations of things you want to do in the next 10 to 15 to 20 years, think about how important your health is for the future. Whether it is for your children, grandchildren, or even for places you want to visit or activities you want to do, you need to be healthy and fit. Regular exercise and maintaining a healthy diet is a lifestyle change, not just a quick fix to lose weight. In order to be healthy and live a long and fulfilling life, continue the improvements you have made in your life and you will see the rewards for many years to come.

Continue reading this daily affirmation to remind yourself that the weight loss goal you have created is also a lifelong existence:

I am successful. I am thin and I am strong. I have overcome many obstacles to get to where I am today. I will continue to live a healthy lifestyle. I will continue to have a positive attitude. I will continue to include my family in my healthy standard of living. I have made the most important decision of my life and I have successfully followed through with it. I have conquered my fears and become a success. I will always strive to be the best I can be and more importantly, I love myself.

Day 31)

You want to lose weight to improve your health. Maybe you're a young mother who desires to see your children get married and produce grandchildren for you or maybe you're middle age worker who wishes to enjoy many years of retirement bliss.

You know that shedding the grease may decrease your chances of getting such maladies as diabetes, heart disease cancer and dementia. You're aware that maintaining a healthy weight will make you feel much better, allow you to play with your children and grandchildren, and ramp up your joy in life. To help you in your quest to achieve your ideal weight, determine what it is and then repeat these affirmations twice daily:

Think on this daily affirmation as a reminder of why thinner and healthier living is so important to you:

I know for a fact that I will weigh X pounds in Y days. I know that I will lose one pound per week. Losing weight won't be difficult because maintaining my health is important to me. I will challenge temptation when it occurs because I deserve to live a long, active life. I deserve to enjoy my grandchildren and a long, productive retirement.

Day 32)

We may blame food for our body size, or at times we may assume that it's our psychology that holds the key to having a slimmer body. Many are the times we suffer through so much just to bring our bodies into that perfect shape that most of us long for. The good news is that you don't have to struggle any more since one thing you need to know is that you're always in control of your body mind and soul.

Reflect on this daily affirmation to remind you of being in full control:

I am in complete control of my body and mind in every way. I cherish my body and would love to help it grow healthier with each passing day.

Day 33)

Everyone wants to have a waist that goes along with his or her hips and body shape. Sometimes our waistline seems to get a bit off proportion from our general physique. Though this might take place naturally giving us little control over the change, it still lowers our self-esteem. This is because we are constantly wondering what people are saying about our body shape. Someone might just be looking at you and you tend to think that they are staring whereas they had no such intention. It creates a feeling of insecurity. At times this hinders us from getting that stylish skirt or suit simply because it has an average waist line and same hip size as yours but your waist line just won't let you, the skirt won't fit at the waist line. To help you get control over your waistline, here is an affirmation that can work for you and your esteem.

Read this daily affirmation when thinking about your waistline seems to bring you to the brink of discouragement:

If I have a diet plan and stick to it, it is easy for me to have control over my middle. That is why I am only taking meals that are healthy and will help me reduce my waistline.

Disclaimers and Legal Stuff

It is the responsibility of each individual person to do their own due diligence regarding the topic of fasting, both starting and ending, juice and water fasts, benefits and disadvantages. Research the Internet, read books, check out various fasting organizations and participate in forums to make the best, most informed choice for **you**. Fast at your own discretion and above all else, don't take any one person's opinion or word for anything. Be smart.

I am not a medical expert and any advice, guidance and observations is from my own research and experience in this area and it is not meant to replace sound, medical advice. Procure the direction of your doctor or healthcare practitioner before you start any fasting regimen.

I touched on it in a previous chapter but it bears mentioning again:

Who should not fast or detoxify:
>   Nursing mothers
>   Pregnant, diabetic women
>   Anorexic or Bulimic individuals
>   Individuals who are too old that their body chemistry can no longer support safe fasting
>   Anyone with severe anemia
>   Some individuals who have a rare, genetic fatty acid deficiency that prevents proper ketosis from occurring
>   Those with porphyria

Who should only fast or detoxify under the supervision of their doctor:

Women who are pregnant
Young children and infants
Individuals with diminished kidney function
Those with Type I diabetes
Someone who might have a serious disease
Individuals who may have a significant fear of fasting but
wish to do so anyway
Individuals using prescriptions should not fast longer
than three days without supervision
Patients who have cancer, a chronic degenerative or
tuberculosis

In no way can I know the specifics about your health and
therefore cannot offer specific advice for your detoxing and
fasting procedures.

Any logos, trademarks, brand names, and graphics are owned by
Integratechs, LLC or used with permission or under license from
a 3rd party.

The informational content within this book is by no means
exhaustive and does not completely explain in depth all
conditions, infections, illnesses, diseases or ailments or their
treatment. Be sure to ask for medical advice from your doctor,
physician or a qualified health care provider about your own
specific needs.

The testimonials or comments in this book are based on my own
fasting and weight loss experiences. You may not have similar
experiences or results.

Using any portion or all of the information contained within this
book is at your own risk. Always cross reference content within

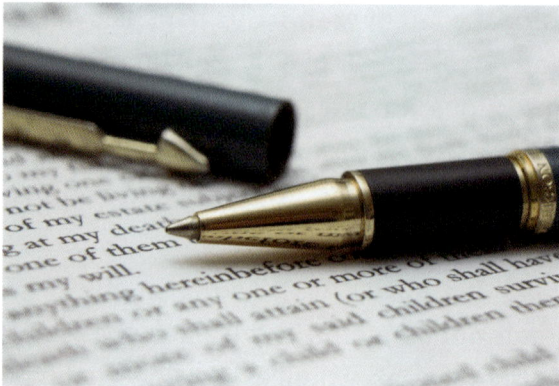

2268397R00057

Printed in Great Britain
by Amazon.co.uk, Ltd.,
Marston Gate.